DOCTOR for the PROSECUTION

DOCTOR
for the
PROSECUTION

A Fighting Surgeon
Takes the Stand

by
Richard Chodoff, M.D.

G. P. PUTNAM'S SONS   New York

The case histories and the pretrial and court testimonies presented in this book are true. In order to protect the identity and privacy of the individuals involved, all names, places and dates have been changed, scenes fictionalized, and any resemblance to persons living or dead is unintentional and coincidental.

The author wishes to thank *The American Lawyer* for permission to reprint an interview of John Bower by Connie Buck in the September 1979 issue of *The American Lawyer*.

Library of Congress Cataloging in Publication Data

Chodoff, Richard.
    Doctor for the prosecution.

    1.Physicians—Malpractice—United States.
I. Title.
KF2905.3.C53   1983   346.7303'32   82-20410
ISBN 0-399-12767-4   347.306332

Printed in the United States of America

For my dear friends
Marvin and Stella Ellin

A physician should expose, without fear or favor, incompetent or corrupt, dishonest or unethical conduct on the part of members of the profession.

—American Medical Association
Principles of Ethics

From the very beginnings of our country, our moral and legal philosophy has been that people should be held accountable for their wrongs and that immunity breeds irresponsibility. Regardless of a person's occupation, if he wrongs another person, he should have to pay for that person's losses.

—Robert E. Cartwright, President,
Trial Lawyers of America

". . . Godammit, I'm asking you to save my life."

"It's not my business to save lives," Doc Daneeka retorted sullenly.

"What is your business?"

"I don't know what my business is. All they ever told me was to uphold the ethics of my profession and never give testimony against another physician."

—Joseph Heller, *Catch-22*

DOCTOR for the PROSECUTION

1

It BEGAN WITH a telephone call in 1968. I remember it was a spring evening, still light and warm outside. The last patient had left, and Mrs. Maxwell, my secretary, already had her jacket on.

"Mr. Waring would like to speak with you, Doctor," she said.

Waring was a lawyer friend of mine, an occasional tennis partner and boating companion. I picked up the phone. "Michael, hello! How's that tennis elbow?"

"Come down to the club next week and I'll show you." He paused. "Actually, Dick, this is a business call."

"Oh? Yours or mine?"

"Both, as it happens." His tone was serious, but still I wasn't prepared for what came next. "I'm calling to ask you to review a hospital file. It involves the death of a youngster, a seventeen-year-old boy."

I remained silent, quite taken aback. I had never been asked to evaluate another surgeon's care of a patient in a case that involved legal action. I was, as Michael well knew, a solid member of the Philadelphia medical community, and, like most of my colleagues, I had been taught early on to obey the profession's unwritten law: Always protect thy colleague.

"You know Hugh Miller?" Michael continued, naming a mutual acquaintance of ours.

"Yes, of course."

11

There was another pause. "Well, it's his son Joey I'm talking about."

"Oh, my God."

Michael sent over Joey Miller's complete medical file that same evening, and I began my study of it then. What I read shocked me. Joey had for some time suffered from peptic-ulcer disease, popularly known as "stomach" ulcer. The ulcer had progressed to the point of perforation, a sudden opening of the intestinal wall that causes spillage into the abdomen. The perforation had, inexplicably, gone unrecognized, and the surgical closure called for was not performed. The failure of Joey's physician to make a simple diagnosis had cost this boy his life. A bright vigorous seventeen-year-old had suffered and died.

I cannot deny that I was thoroughly shaken. This was, after all, the hospital I practiced in, these were the physicians I worked with. I too had children, and I remember thinking to myself, My God, suppose this had been Bill or Mary that they killed.

I called Michael Waring and told him exactly what I thought. Joey Miller's case was a medical tragedy.

"I'm sending you my report, Michael. To tell you the truth, if I hadn't seen the files I don't know whether I would have believed it. Poor Hugh. I kept thinking of my own kids."

"I know. It really hits close to home, doesn't it?" Michael said. "If the case comes to court will you testify?"

It was, of course, the logical and inevitable next question. All the same, I wasn't ready for it.

"Dick? Are you there?"

"Yes, of course. Listen, Michael, you know what you're asking me to do. I don't think I can give you an answer now. It's too big a question. I'm going to need some time."

I put down the receiver very slowly and gently. It was the gesture of a disturbed and confused man, and I knew it. If I agreed to Michael's request I would be involved in a malpractice suit against my fellows. I was under no illusion about the attitude of the medical profession toward a doctor who would testify that a colleague had harmed or killed a patient. Like a medieval brotherhood of knights, physicians gird their loins, lower their lances and form a protective ring about their errant comrade, doing their best to make certain that his professional reputation remains unsullied. I would be considered a turncoat. The price of rebellion against the established order would be high, the risks great and the reprisals inevitable.

I spent that weekend in the usual way between hospital and home, but I remember it only for a demanding and unceasing inner dialogue. Before I could answer Michael's question I had to be able to understand some of my own.

My father, my two brothers and my son were all doctors. If I agreed to be a witness for the plaintiff, would I be offending not only a professional tradition but a family one? Yet was it a tradition worth upholding? I had been carefully taught, in one way or another, that "mistakes" happen and a fellow doctor should be forgiven and protected. The majority of surgeons, the group with which I am most familiar, are honest, ethical and competent. And they err, as do I, but these are not errors of neglect or improper medical care. I know from my own experience that the greatest punishment that can be inflicted upon a surgeon who has inadvertently caused suffering to a patient is his self-recrimination. But are self-blame and silent breast-beating to be considered adequate compensation when real damage has been done? Surely it was time for me to define "mistake" more clearly. What had happened to Joey Miller was carelessness too extreme to qualify as a mistake.

My dialogue was not without its mea culpas. In my thirty years as a practicing surgeon I had, of course, seen many other examples of carelessness and negligence. Why had I waited so long to allow myself full awareness; to recognize the plight of an injured patient or bereaved family? Had my compassion been aroused only because the man involved in this medical "mistake" was my friend?

My thoughts continued in this way. I suppose, in a sense, I was conducting my own trial. Could I in good conscience continue to be a part of this conspiracy of silence, to uphold the image of my profession as a group incapable of wrong? My more pragmatic self demanded to know if I could afford to have a conscience. How much would my practice suffer? For surely some of my outraged colleagues would stop referring patients to me. My surgical practice was an interesting and busy one. I was at this time on the staff of Jefferson Medical College and the Albert Einstein Medical Center in Philadelphia and of suburban Haverford Hospital, which, with a small group of doctors, I had helped found in 1958. Was I really willing to put all this in jeopardy?

The word "malpractice" had always been as abhorrent to me as it was to most other doctors. Yet, with young Joey's death some floodgate deep within me had finally given way and waves of long-repressed doubt and guilt washed over me. I recalled my discomfort on the occasions I'd seen negligent or incompetent surgery, how I was always left with the uneasy feeling that I should have done something, or at least said something. I compared myself to the Nazi Party member who, after the war, asked forgiveness because he was only a "little man" who obeyed orders and was too frightened to protest.

I continued to brood in this way for four or five days, visited by the past the way a man is when he comes to a sudden turning point in his life. I took restless walks around Philadelphia, revisiting Pine Street where I grew up, or, because ships and sailing have been a lifelong passion, I would wander down along the Delaware River at Penn's Landing. I thought I was seeking a moment's peace, but what I was looking for, of course, was the courage to make a difficult decision.

My father was fond of observing that for a man to get safely over middle age was like Hannibal crossing the Alps. Well, I had not reached my sixtieth peak without a few certain scars. There is the literal one on the right side of my neck, the result of a partial thyroidectomy and radical neck dissection for cancer of the thyroid; a mark that serves to remind me of the apprehension and pain my surgical patients feel.

And there is the figurative scar that mars the conscience, the guilt of my contribution to an unsuccessful first marriage. When I was a resident at Philadelphia's Mount Sinai Hospital, I met a lovely nurse named Dean Owens and we became good friends. Inevitably, our friendship turned into romance, and in 1938 we married. Dean was a bright woman, a good and honest one, but I was not mature enough to yield, without considerable resentment, to the restrictions of marriage. I wanted my marital comfort, yet I balked at giving up my carefree bachelor life. In 1943 our son, Bill, was born in Paris, Texas, where I was one of the surgeons at the Army station hospital. We adopted our daughter, Mary, ten years later, but it was a vain and unfair hope to think that children could strengthen a foundering marriage. For years Dean and I had been inhabiting some kind of bleak emotional wasteland, very close to divorce but never quite taking that final step.

Behind the memories that kept crowding into my head I could hear Michael say, "If the case comes to court will you testify?" He had put that loaded question to me casually, but his voice had been as tense as mine when I said I needed time to decide. And time I did need, for, not surprisingly, my search for the answer was leading me all the way back to my childhood; to my mother's earnest belief in the innate goodness of mankind and to my father's practical proof of her doctrine. He was an old-time general practitioner, not the most learned of men, perhaps, but a compassionate doctor who willingly attended his patients at any hour of the day or night.

I thought about the afternoons I used to spend in my father's waiting room when I was a child. Many of his patients were Italian, and I became more adept at greeting people in Italian than in my own language. As soon as the patients left I would run to the bookcase and take down the books of anatomy, urology, gynecology. And I'd sit hidden behind the big leather chair, puzzling over the illustrations until it was suppertime.

My father's working hours were long, for he would never refuse a call from a patient. I have one particularly cherished memory of him, clear and vivid, although I was only a small child at the time. In 1918 there was a catastrophic influenza epidemic; the illness was sudden and overwhelming, the death rate was high, and there was no specific treatment for it. My father would start out in the early morning with a long list of patients to see; at each stop he would be besieged by neighbors with influenza in the family. He would come home late at night, completely exhausted but ready to go again by dawn.

When the depression began in 1929, not only were many of his calls made without charge but I later found out that he used to leave money for his patients to buy food. When I myself became a doctor, people hearing me paged would stop me in the hospital corridors to inquire whether I was related to Dr. Louis Chodoff. When I said that I was his son, I was overwhelmed by loving words for the man who had been their physician and friend.

A profound respect for humanity was, I think, the great bond between my parents. My mother was a beautiful dark-haired woman. She dressed elegantly but simply; was soft-spoken yet eloquent. Brought up as a militant atheist, she taught my two brothers and me the absolute importance of love and decency toward our fellow men.

My father was not an intellectual. His interests did not lie in music and literature as my mother's did. His greatest love was gambling; he would bet on baseball games, horseraces, even the gender of a baby about to be born. Each Saturday he would take part in a crap game at one of the hotels known to be a gathering place for doctors. Since most of the police force in Philadelphia, especially in the center city, were either friends or patients of the gambling doctors, the games were never disturbed. Although my mother was fully aware of my father's activities, he never admitted his losses to her but always bragged about his infrequent winnings. He was a tall, handsome man with the sort of waxed mustache that doctors sported in the early 1900s. A true bon vivant, he always wore a white carnation in his lapel. I remember how touched I was at his funeral when a lady whom he had known for a long time, perhaps quite well, dropped a white carnation on the casket as it was lowered into the grave.

My mother was the charming hostess of one of Philadelphia's most interesting salons. The street that we lived on was known as the doctors' row. There were about twelve to fifteen doctors' offices in the block, but I think ours was the only house that had entire theater and ballet companies coming to parties. My mother's guests also included members of the Philadelphia Orchestra, newspapermen and artists. The conversations my brothers and I listened to, and later took part in, covered a broad range of interests, and so I grew up used to a constant exchange of ideas. Our library was voluminous, and before I finished high school I had avidly read my way through most of the classics.

But drawn though I was to the world of literature, there never seemed to be any question in my mind that I would go on to medical school. In fact, my studies really began when I was still in my teens and supplemented a small allowance by assisting my father with tonsillectomies in his office on Sunday mornings. I was the anesthetist, first assistant, nurse, orderly and porter. I became adept at holding a separate instrument with each finger while at the same time administering open-drop ether, our only anesthetic agent and fortunately for me a very safe one to give. After the tonsils and adenoids had been removed I would carry the children to a spare bedroom on the second floor and put them to bed, where they would rest until their parents took them home in the evening. Once in a while a child would begin to bleed, and I would have the fearsome task of bringing him back down to the office and anesthetizing him again so that my father could suture the bleeding area in his tonsillar bed. It was a tribute to my father's skill, and our amazing good luck, that we never lost a patient.

My seventeenth summer I briefly ran away to sea. Inspired by the books of Joseph Conrad, my cousin Charles and I went to the waterfront office of Shanghai Johnson, a well-known shipping agent. He told us that there was an oil tanker leaving almost immediately for the West Coast via the Panama Canal and that if we wanted the mess-boy jobs we would have to hurry to Petty's Island, in the Delaware, where the ship was berthed. We decided not to battle against the lure of the sea, and off we went to Petty's Island to sign on for that long trip to Panama.

Medical school, internship, surgical residency . . . such an unexpected assortment of memories come back to me. In the summer of 1933 I began, as my father had done before me, a twenty-seven-month rotating internship at Jefferson Hospital. Spending three-month periods on each service, I moved through a variety of medical specialties, learning about each. The atmosphere of hospitals was somewhat different then. There was less competition and more feeling of fellowship and cooperation. Life was simpler and kinder.

Yet even in those early days of our medical careers, I noticed a disturbing pose of omnipotence among my peers. How the lack of a little human tact and empathy could destroy the doctor–patient relationship, was unforgettably illustrated to me by a fellow intern who had been an academic leader in his medical school. At the end of one of our rotation periods he took over the patients I had been responsible for. One of them, an older woman named Mrs. Bellamy, to whom I had been giving a daily intravenous injection, I found packing the day after services changed. She was determined, against all medical counsel, to sign out of the hospital. In tears of fright and indignation she explained that while my colleague had been giving her the injection he had casually observed, "You know, Mrs. Bellamy, I could kill you in thirty seconds if I gave you this too fast."

But if my awareness of awkward medical attitudes and situations began at this time, so, too, did my acceptance of them. In my subsequent two years as chief surgical resident at Mount Sinai Hospital I found ways to absorb the disillusion I met on discovering that doctors with the greatest reputations are not necessarily the best ones. The eminent physician under whom I served was, I soon realized, indecisive, unsure of his own capabilities, and quick to compromise in order to maintain his reputation as a safe surgeon. This "safety" was in great part due to performing inadequate surgery on patients whose cure rate would have been far higher with more radical procedures. But this, of course, also involved a higher percentage of morbidity and mortality, which my chief did not wish to risk.

We residents and interns tended on the whole to overlook the deficiencies of the staff members, accepting them as part of the human condition. If we encountered health-endangering substandard care, either we didn't recognize it or else we adopted the profession's prevailing attitude that "the doctor had done his best." I never really attempted to differentiate between the unavoidable complications that arose during conscientious care of a patient and those problems that resulted from negligence. Like my fellows I paid homage to the physicians "mistake." I also learned to smile at the "foibles" none of us ever dared criticize, to stand quietly in the respectful retinue of a prominent internist who on his rounds would invariably listen to the patient's heart with a stethoscope whose earpieces still lay around his neck.

At the end of my residency I started private practice as a surgeon. Since I couldn't afford an office of my own, my father generously shared his with me. Patients were few at first, but referrals slowly increased and by the end of the first year I was almost making a living. More importantly, I was beginning to experience the fulfillment of a surgeon's life. My time was divided between my practice, ward service at Mount Sinai and the surgical clinic at Jefferson, where I was fortunate enough to work with Dr. Howard Bradshaw, one of the pioneer chest surgeons. We did what research we could with our rather rudimentary equipment, but if our techniques were crude in the beginning we had the satisfaction of seeing each year bring improvements and higher survival rates.

Because of my work in the surgical treatment of tuberculosis I was appointed visiting surgeon to White Haven Sanitorium. In the late thirties and early forties there were no drugs for tuberculosis. The accepted treatment was rest and, when indicated, the collapse of the diseased areas of the lung. Once a month I would drive up to the sanitorium with an anesthesiologist. There, in the isolation of the Pocono Mountains, we would operate, removing ribs over diseased lungs, dividing the adhesions that interfered with the lung's collapse, from morning until evening.

Was I now to turn my back on medical tradition, to act upon my conviction that a colleague had done an immense harm? A strange pattern of memories came back to me, with certain scenes in sharp focus. There was, for instance, the Army. After being stationed in Texas at Camp Maxey I was assigned chief of the general surgical section of a 1,000-bed hospital in England.

Our surgical-department head, a genial and pleasant man from the South, had become a Fellow of the College of Surgeons, largely, I think, on the basis of the minor surgical procedures he had performed. As severely wounded men were brought to us, many requiring major chest or abdominal surgery, he would invariably say to me in his casual Southern accent, "Would you like to do this one?" It soon became apparent that he was incapable of doing major surgery.

One evening a young man with multiple shell fragment abdominal wounds was brought to us. His condition was precarious. He was draining large amounts of intestinal fluid, and it was clear that without immediate surgery he would die. The procedure in those days was a formidable one and carried a large mortality risk. Still, it had to be attempted. I hurried to tell my chief about this patient and was stunned to hear him say that as the patient would almost surely die if operated upon, he would not permit me to operate. "We don't want any surgical deaths on our record," he said. I argued with him, but I got nowhere. Time was running out and I told him that if he didn't operate, or permit me to, I would call the surgical consultant for our entire area; that I would present the problem to him and let him make the final decision. As this would surely precipitate an inspection unflattering to my chief, he reluctantly gave me permission to operate. I did, and the patient survived to go home.

I returned to practice in 1946 after four years in the Army, the last of which was spent at Valley Forge General Hospital, where I was in charge of the general surgical section. Some of the fearsome mutilations I saw in young men who should have been destined for a peaceful, rewarding life horrified me. It seemed to me that there had to be better ways of settling international disputes than the murderous methods we used.

When I returned to Jefferson Hospital I was an attending surgeon on the wards. This involved making rounds with the residents and the medical students, and because they were always full of questions I found it an invigorating experience. But for me the most fascinating aspect of teaching had to do with surgery itself, and nothing was quite as rewarding as those days when I scrubbed in the operating room to assist and teach surgical technique to the senior resident.

I was also working at Mount Sinai Hospital at this time, and eventually I became one of the attending surgeons at the then Southern Division of the Albert Einstein Medical Center. Here too I had the opportunity of helping to train many residents, some of whom came to us from foreign countries.

Although I have never been the back-slapping, gregarious kind of person who achieves influence in the inner circles of organized medicine, I made advances in my surgical work, my practice grew and I became a respectable member of the establishment. But even then I knew there was much I chose to shield my gaze from: the unnecessary operations performed only for the fees involved; post-operative care that sometimes made me shudder; and careless, inept surgery done by unscrupulous men. More than once I was confronted with evidence of the latter. There was a Mrs. Charles who was sent to me with typical gall bladder symptoms. She had been admitted to one of the large teaching hospitals in Philadelphia with a diagnosis of gallstones and was operated upon by a well-known surgeon for removal of the gall bladder. A short time later Mrs. Charles's symptoms recurred. She went back to the same surgeon and was X-rayed, and gallstones were seen once again. She underwent surgery a second time. When I X-rayed Mrs. Charles I found still another gall bladder containing gallstones. It was quite difficult for me to understand how a woman whose gall bladder had been taken out twice could still have one full of stones. More difficult yet to explain this to Mrs. Charles. Finally she permitted me to convince her that she needed surgery a third time, and I admitted her to the hospital. When I operated I found that Mrs. Charles had what is known as an intraheptic gall bladder, one that is not visible below the liver but is embedded within the liver substance. Obviously the previous surgeon had not been competent enough to handle the rather difficult technical procedure. I took out the gall bladder and assured Mrs. Charles that she would never have to have it removed again.

But despite such disillusionment I continued to believe that medicine, especially surgery, was the noblest of professions. I counseled myself to mind my own business and concentrate on being a good and conscientious surgeon. I studied current medical journals, attended surgical meetings, and visited hospitals abroad whenever I could.

Believing as I did in the medical profession, I went on suppressing my doubts about a doctrine that compelled physicians to protect each other. I held at bay my secret concern that there was no such protection for the patients who were damaged by negligent doctors or by substandard hospital care. I continued to compromise with my conscience by extending help in other directions. In 1965 I volunteered to spend a month in a hospital in the interior of Malaysia for Medico-Care, an organization which supplied specialists on a rotating basis to hospitals in remote areas of the world. I was assigned a small jungle hospital in a town called Kuala Lipis, where I was surgeon, urologist, orthopedist, gynecologist, whatever was needed. It was a challenging time, and I was frequently taken by surprise.

The first patient I operated upon, a young woman of about thirty, had obstructive jaundice. I assumed that gallstones had migrated into the bile duct, had become stuck and were causing bile blockage. I operated on her, firmly expecting to find a large stone in her common bile duct. When I opened the duct, I was amazed and horrified to find instead several round worms obstructing the duct, creatures about sixteen to eighteen inches long and thick as my finger. This was only the first of many similar cases.

The hospital library was a very meager one, but fortunately there was an ancient book of operative surgery among the half-dozen volumes. This I was enormously grateful for when a ten-year-old Aborigine girl was brought to me. She was an intelligent and charming child with a cleft palate, a split in the roof of her mouth, which badly interfered with her speech. This was a condition in which I had no experience at all. I found a description, though very crude, in the old surgery book, and decided to operate. To our mutual delight she had an excellent result.

I began to see that these random memories were leading me to an inevitable decision. In each of them I recognized something of the way I felt about myself, and about medicine. I didn't know what to call it. A restlessness in my spirit, a stubbornness and determination, and a kind of elation. Finally my mind was made up. I called Michael Waring and told him that, yes, if Joey Miller's case came to court I would testify. Later the case was settled out of court, and for all my soul-searching I could not deny a certain sense of relief.

2

ONE DAY ABOUT a month later, a morning when several operations were scheduled, I arrived at the hospital earlier than usual.

"I've made coffee, Doctor," Mrs. Maxwell greeted me with her special brand of efficiency. After years of working with me she often knew my mind before I did.

"Exactly what I want, Virginia. Thanks."

"And a Miss Stone called. I told her you'd be in soon."

"Fine." As I spoke the phone rang and I took the call myself.

"Dr. Chodoff?"

"Yes?"

"My name is Paula Stone. I'm a friend of Michael Waring." It was a young woman's voice, low and pleasant. "I wonder if it would be possible to see you today."

"Well, it's a pretty busy day for me . . . but if it's urgent you could come in late this afternoon. Just a minute and I'll have my secretary give you an appointment."

"Doctor, wait, please." Miss Stone had the merest hint of amusement in her voice. "I should tell you it's a different sort of urgency."

"Oh? I see." As Michael had sent her, I ought to have realized that much.

"Well, Mrs. Maxwell will give you a time. We try not to discriminate in urgencies here."

"That's what I'd hoped."

My day was made even longer than I had anticipated by an emergency appendectomy on an old girl of eighty-eight. She had a slight respiratory problem coming out of the anesthesia, and I wanted to stay close by until she made it out of Recovery and down to her own room. It was nearly six o'clock when I got back to my office, and, to tell the truth, I'd forgotten about that morning's mysterious phone call.

"Your appointment's here, Doctor," Mrs. Maxwell said. "The young woman who called this morning."

"Oh—right. Of course. Send her in, please."

A slender dark-haired young woman whom I guessed to be in her late twenties came into my office.

"I'm Paula Stone," she said, reaching across the desk to give my hand a firm businesslike shake. "I know this wasn't the most convenient time for you to see me, Doctor. I really do appreciate it."

"My pleasure," I said, and to my surprise I really meant it. There was an alertness, a rare intelligence that animated this young woman's face. And a very beautiful face it was—white, nearly translucent skin, large green eyes and a wide generous smile.

"I'll get right to the point, Doctor," she said, with a direct forthright look that made me realize I was not the only one making appraisals. "I'm told you're a man who isn't afraid of the truth."

"You present me with an interesting conundrum, Miss Stone. Only a man who can deny that is unafraid."

She gave a husky laugh, but her eyes held a very sober expression. "As you've probably guessed, Doctor, I'm here to ask you to review a file."

I sat up in my chair, straight and rather stiffly. "No, in fact, I didn't quite guess that."

If my visitor noticed my sudden discomfort she ignored it. "Let's go back to the beginning, then. You see, I'm a medical-legal consultant, and when Michael told me about you, a respected, first-rate surgeon who's really concerned about what's happening to the injured patient—"

I held up my hand. "Wait, please, Miss Stone. I am very concerned, it's true, but before you go any further let me explain

24

that when I agreed to review that file for Michael, well, that was a very special case."

She raised a critical eyebrow. "Aren't they all? I don't think I understand."

"Let me put it this way. I did a great deal of mulling things over before I decided to testify for the plaintiff, and I'd have done it gladly, but, as Michael may have told you, the case was settled out of court." I paused, wondering how to phrase my complex feelings. "I suppose what I'm trying to say, Miss Stone, is that my primary concern is over my own patients, not other doctors'. Of course, I'm very aware of the problems that arise from malpractice. Personally, I feel the time's come for serious changes in the way the medical profession handles these things. But—"

She interrupted me with a rueful look. "You don't have to say anything more, Dr. Chodoff. I'm very familiar with that particular 'but.' The defendant doctor has no problem finding an expert witness. They'll come in droves to protect a colleague even when they privately agree he's guilty. But just try to find a physician to protect some poor unknown patient. Or the surviving family. Well, thanks anyway, Doctor." She stood up to go with a polite proud smile that didn't quite hide her resignation and disappointment.

"No need to jump up like a jack-in-the-box, Miss Stone," I said, waving her back to her chair as I might have done one of my students. "I just wanted you to know my general outlook. My particular feelings will depend on the case. Now why don't you tell me exactly what and who this is all about."

Paula Stone sat down again and told me about the case. She spoke briefly and precisely, only her intense expression betraying the obvious concern she felt for the widow plaintiff. "It happened in a small town—out in Arizona. A young man named Tom Wilson, about thirty-two, was in an automobile accident. He was thrown hard against the steering wheel. Apparently he had been drinking, and the police took him down to the jail. Two hours later he was having such severe abdominal pains they had to transfer him to the hospital. Thirty-six hours later he was dead. He left a family—wife, two babies—and no money. The young widow went to a lawyer, a good man named Edward Baker. Michael knows him, by the way.

Anyway, Baker feels certain it was a case of negligence, but he can't find a surgical expert willing to stick his neck out even to the extent of reviewing the case."

"And what do you think?"

"Well, I'm not qualified to give a medical opinion, of course, but I think Baker is right. If I hadn't believed malpractice or negligence was definitely involved, I'd have sent the file right back—which is what I do most of the time."

There was no mistaking either her honesty or her dismay over this case. "Okay, I'll read the file, but please understand that doesn't mean I'm saying I'll be your witness. If I think there truly is negligence, well, we'll talk about it then. Meanwhile, may I ask you a personal question?"

"Yes, of course," my visitor replied, her hands folded in her lap like a prim schoolgirl.

"How did you become so interested in medicine?"

"I suppose I just always was, even as a child. After college I went to medical school for a couple of years—as long as the money held out, and then I had to quit. So I started working in related areas. First I did a lot of editing for two National Institutes of Health magazines, then I compiled an extensive medical brief for an attorney who had the first Thalidomide case in this country. It was he who first suggested that I become a medical-legal consultant."

"Meaning precisely?"

She laughed. "You have a very scientific approach, Doctor. Well, let me try to be more explicit. Lawyers send me medical files, and if I think there's any question of malpractice I'll ask a board-certified specialist to review the case. If the expert feels there has indeed been a departure from the normal standard of care, he'll write a detailed summary of his opinion. Then I start going to the libraries, digging out every bit of pertinent surgical literature, and eventually I send a compilation of everything back to the lawyer. There," she said, smiling as she stopped to catch her breath.

"I take it you're always hired by the plaintiff lawyers?"

She shook her head. "Not at all. I've done work for the defense. And a certain amount of work in private liability cases. Industrial firms, you know, that sort of thing."

"But that's not exactly where your heart is, is it?" I gave her a look as direct as her own, and she lowered her eyes.

"Well, naturally one feels more . . . involved when it's a question of being able to help people who've got all the cards stacked against them."

"Like the young widow in Arizona?"

She colored faintly. "I'm no young romantic idealist, Dr. Chodoff, believe me. It's a rough world out there—and I have few illusions. I run a business, not a charity organization." She made her voice brisk. "I'm paid for the time and work I put into a case like this. As, by the way, you'd be if you agreed to review the file and be an expert witness. Let's just say this happens to be my profession and that—like you—I'm very committed to my work."

Mrs. Maxwell rang me at this point on the interoffice phone. "It's almost eight o'clock, Doctor."

"Good lord, I'm sorry, Virginia. I had no idea."

"You never even had lunch today, Doctor, did you?"

"I'll make up for it at dinner."

Miss Stone was standing, ready to leave, and somehow it seemed the most natural thing in the world to suggest that we continue our conversation over dinner—something we are still doing, as I write this, twelve years later. For there was no denying the strong attraction we felt for each other at that first meeting. It is, I believe, a not uncommon characteristic of true love that it sometimes comes into existence full-blown and deeply rooted.

So at any rate it was with Paula and me. I regained with her something I'd lost in my youth—the ease and comfort of being with a kindred spirit. In the weeks and months that followed, over long dinners at my favorite little Italian restaurant, in crowded theater lobbies and on the deck of my sailboat, we continued the dialogue that had begun in my office. Whether we were discussing the excitement of medicine, the anguish of malpractice or a shared passion for reading, I found in Paula the kind of humanity, the deep compassion I had not encountered outside my parents' home. That there was a considerable difference in our ages, thirty years to be exact, neither of us seemed to notice. A profound respect for each other's work and a camaraderie based on mutual interests spanned the difference in our ages to unite us in a deep love. At the end of that year when my divorce became final, Paula and I were married.

In the fall of 1970, some eighteen months after I reviewed Tom Wilson's file, I went to Arizona to appear in court for the first time as an expert witness for the plaintiff.

The facts of this case were distressingly simple. On a Friday night Mr. Wilson drove his Volkswagen bus into the rear end of a car stopped ahead of him at an intersection. He was thrown against the steering wheel with such force that the steering wheel crumpled. It was a more or less typical "steering-wheel injury." At the jail the police became so alarmed when they found their prisoner bent double and writhing with abdominal pain that they transferred him to the local hospital, where the defendant, Dr. Carson, saw him for the first time. The tentative diagnosis was a "possible abdominal injury."

A review of Tom Wilson's hospital chart showed that the initial physical examination had been woefully incomplete. Dr. Carson's indifference went so far as to include an order left for a soft diet, absolutely forbidden when an intestinal injury is suspected. Though the purpose of the patient's admission on Friday night was to keep him under close observation, he was not seen again until nine o'clock on Saturday morning, fourteen hours later. At that time Dr. Carson said that Tom was still "hung over," and he did not bother to examine him. The patient was not seen again until 7:30 P.M. that day, when he was dying. In spite of the resuscitation attempts then made by Dr. Carson's partner, Dr. Randolph, Tom Wilson died at 7:40 P.M.

Mrs. Wilson, who had spent most of her husband's last day at his bedside, described him as in extreme pain, his skin cold and clammy, his pulse weak—accurate observations of a man dying of hemorrhagic shock and peritonitis. When an autopsy was performed the following day, the pathologist found Mr. Wilson's abdomen filled with feces and blood from a complete tear of the small bowel, obviously incurred at the time of the accident.

This type of injury, when there has been no penetration of the abdominal wall, as in bullet or knife wounds, is known as blunt abdominal trauma, and it is vital that the patient be examined frequently, as there is always the possibility of internal injuries. There ought to have been X-ray and laboratory studies—all the parameters that help tell a doctor what is happening to his patient. But most important, the attending surgeon ought to have kept him under close observation, for the condition of such a patient can change from hour to hour and an operation might become necessary at any time. The failure of Dr. Carson to do any of this made Tom Wilson's death inevitable.

I felt I had no choice but to agree to be the plaintiff's expert witness. Though I was strengthened by Paula's warm approval of my decision, I confess I felt more than a little uneasy when the time actually came to go to court.

My trip to Clayton, Arizona, was more than a geographical move; it was going from operating room to courtroom, from respectable member of the establishment to maverick surgeon. I can't pretend that I did not find this new role confusing and frightening. As the plane neared its destination I wondered what I had got myself into. Would I actually see the doctor I was testifying against? Would his lawyer attack me? Was I going to be able to withstand the pressures? I reminded myself that there was no way that they could justify what had happened to Tom Wilson. A young man dies needlessly; his wife is left alone, penniless, with two small children. All this I told myself, but at the same time I was aware that a few years ago I would have understood the physicians who said, Why, that son of a bitch is going to testify against another doctor. He ought to lose his position. He ought to be ostracized. Nobody should refer cases to him.

It's never an easy thing, I suppose, to break with the tradition you've been brought up in. I really didn't have much idea of what was actually going to happen. I didn't quite know how I was going to behave. Whether I was going to be scared. Whether I was going to be articulate. Whether I was going to stutter and stammer. Whether the adrenaline would come in sufficient quantity to let me be persuasive or whether I would be a backward witness who would do more harm than good.

It was almost a relief when the plane finally landed in a small airport near Clayton. Edward Baker, a tall, rather thin young man in his late thirties, was waiting for me. He had an open, friendly face with a quick smile and sober gray eyes magnified by his glasses.

"Welcome to Arizona," he said, shaking my hand.

"I guess you're the only one who is going to say that," I told him with a nervous smile.

"Oh, no, there's my client," he said, laughing, and I knew we were going to get along fine.

We spent the next day at Ed's office preparing for the trial. We had a lot to learn from each other and not much time to do it. I had to direct his line of questioning so that he could elicit the proper medical information from his witnesses. He had to teach me a new vocabulary, how to think in words that a jury of laymen would understand.

"I don't know whether you've any idea how relieved and grateful my client was to know you were coming out here," Ed told me that night at dinner. "It's pretty near impossible to find a well-qualified surgeon like you who will risk going to bat for the patient."

"I suppose that's what finally got through to me," I replied. "A little late in life, perhaps, but nevertheless here I am."

"I wish more doctors could see that their compassion for the patient has to extend beyond the consulting room." Ed took off his glasses and gave me his grave myopic stare. "No matter what the profession's wish may be, malpractice is a subject that won't go on being ignored much longer."

"Let's hope, for everybody's sake, and I mean my colleagues as well as their patients, that you're right."

"By the way," Ed said, "Mrs. Wilson is anxious to meet you and I thought you might have a few questions you want to ask her. I told her we'd stop by after dinner." He folded his napkin. "It's a damn shame, you know. She's a nice young woman, and I don't know how she's going to manage to keep her family together if we don't win the case."

"She doesn't work?"

"No, the kids are too little to be left. Anyway, there aren't that many jobs around here. Especially for somebody without special training." He took off his glasses again. "I hope I'm doing the right thing for her, Dick. You're not the only one who's feeling nervous about this trial. The insurance company offered a settlement of thirty thousand and I turned it down. I wanted to get her at least fifty."

"My God, I would hope so."

"Sure, but you have to remember where we are. Now I keep worrying, what if I lose the case?"

"I just don't see how, from a medical point of view, that would be possible. The man was killed by negligence. What kind of jury will there be?"

"Just ordinary local folks. I'll be surprised if they turn in a large verdict, but I've got to try. A lot will depend on how they react to you. Now, the judge is okay. No great shakes, but he's a decent man. We'll get a fair trial. The trouble is, of course, the usual one. Every other doctor in town is going to testify for the defense. They'll swear to anything in order to defend their own. You're my only medical testimony." He smiled. "It's a case of David against Goliath."

We drove through the town of Clayton and out to a housing development and pulled up in front of a small yellow frame house, differing from all the others only in its color. It was one of those prefabricated jobs that could be picked up and moved around the country almost as easily as a trailer. There was a patch of lawn with an abandoned tricycle, a sandbox and a sparse unyielding flower garden that made a border around the house.

I don't know what I'd been expecting, but I was surprised by the diminutive pretty young woman who opened the door. She was fragile, far too pale, with large black eyes startling in their depth. She held a sleeping baby in her arms and with a shy apologetic smile motioned for us to come in.

"I'm just getting my little girl to bed. Please make yourselves comfortable. There's coffee on that tray over there. I'll only be a minute."

I followed Baker into the small but well-furnished and tidy living room. There was a piano in the corner with a series of photographs on its top. I walked over and looked at the young laughing face of Tom Wilson. His clear blue eyes seemed to look into my own for an instant, and I felt the frustration of this needless death more keenly because now the deceased had a face. In the next photograph he was holding a baby high in the air, proud as a peacock. There was a birthday picture, Christmas, a summer day at the beach—a whole life left sitting on top of the piano.

"That was Tom," Mrs. Wilson said, coming up behind me. She knew, of course, that I would know who it was, but it made her feel better to say it. "We had good times together." She was miles away for several long moments, and then with an effort she brought herself back and straightened a few of the pictures. "I really appreciate what you're doing Dr. Chodoff." She was obviously fighting to keep her emotions in control, and her voice was low and unsteady. "Mr. Baker said you might have some questions about Tom. But excuse me, I'm afraid I'm not being a very good hostess." For a moment embarrassment brought color to her cheeks. "Are you sure you won't have coffee or something?"

I took a cup of coffee and sat down on the bright chintz sofa, but the only questions I could bring myself to ask were about her two little girls. It was, of course, the only safe subject, the one I knew would bring a real smile to her face.

"I think Dr. Chodoff has a few facts he'd like to check with you, Clara," Ed finally said, pointing the conversation in its necessary direction.

"I've read your deposition, so this really isn't essential, you know," I told her. "There are just a few details I'm curious about, that's all."

"It's okay. I understand," she said.

I hesitated. "I believe you said your husband already had severe pain when he entered the hospital for observation on Friday night?"

"He was doubled over in agony, Doctor. I mean he just couldn't keep himself straightened out, the pain was so bad."

"Can you remember the first thing they did for him at the hospital?"

"They didn't do anything." There was a brief flash of anger in Mrs. Wilson's dark eyes. "Nothing, nothing at all. They just kept saying we'd have to wait for Dr. Carson to come and that he'd be there soon but he didn't show up for another two hours at least."

"And after the doctor got there," Ed Baker prompted, "What did he do for Tom?"

"Well, still nothing. Dr. Carson didn't think there was any problem. He said Tom was going to be just fine." She bit her lip and turned her head away. "I'm sorry," she murmured, her voice barely audible. "I promised myself I wasn't going to, you know, carry on . . ."

"You're not, my dear," I said, patting her shoulder awkwardly. "And I'm the one who's sorry, asking you to talk about these things. I think we should call it a night now, don't you, Ed?"

"No, I'm fine, I really am," Mrs. Wilson said. "And I want to be helpful. Please go on, Dr. Chodoff."

"Well, I'll be as brief as I can, then. How did your husband look to you the morning after the accident, do you remember?"

She nodded. "Sometimes I pray that God will let me forget. I mean I still have nightmares about it. That's when I knew, I guess, that morning, how really bad off he was. He had this ghastly look, this kind of pallor, you know, and he kept groaning and saying he'd rather be dead than go on suffering like that from the pain in his stomach."

"And what explanation did Dr. Carson give you about your husband's condition at that point?"

"He never explained anything. He wasn't even there then. And the nurses, all they ever said was that I shouldn't be so nervous, that Tom was going to be okay."

I cleared my throat. I hated having to remind her of this tragic sequence of events. "When was it you first noticed the bruise on your husband's abdomen?"

"I think it was Saturday morning. It might have been there before, but I hadn't looked. He was in terrible pain, nothing seemed to be helping, and I was straightening his bed covers when I noticed a deep reddish-purple bruise. I rang for the nurse and I pointed it out to her and asked if that wasn't what was causing Tom such pain. She said that the doctor was aware of it and I shouldn't keep worrying so much."

I turned to Ed. "Strange that the only record of the bruise I've come across is in the autopsy report. People don't bruise after they're dead, you know."

"Sorry, my dear," I said to Mrs. Wilson. "Now, tell me, they kept sending in soft-diet trays, is that right?"

"Yes, but he couldn't even look at food, he felt so awful." Her dark eyes filled with tears. "Nobody would listen to me about anything. It was like they were dismissing Tom's pain and everything as part of a hangover." She glanced up at me. "I suppose you know he'd been drinking?"

I nodded. "A man's care in the hospital doesn't depend upon sobriety," I said, but I wondered if perhaps she wasn't right. "Was there anything else you noticed?"

"Later on, in the afternoon, his skin began to get kind of cold and clammy. I was sitting by the bed, holding his hand, and suddenly I couldn't even hardly feel his pulse."

"Did you tell the nurses this?" Ed asked.

"Oh, yes. I got really scared and I ran out in the corridor calling for help. The nurses, they tried to calm me down and they said a doctor would come and look at Tom." Mrs. Wilson took a deep shuddering breath. "But by then it was too late."

The tears she had been holding back all evening began to fall. She wept silently, but nevertheless, in that remarkable way children have of picking up emotional vibrations, her small daughter got out of bed and came to the living-room door.

"Mommy?" she called hesitatingly. Her eyes, big and dark as her mother's, were also filled with tears.

With two grandchildren of my own, I was not at a total loss in this situation, and soon not only the little girl was laughing at my grandfatherly nonsense but Mrs. Wilson too. It was a nervous laugh on her part, to be sure, no more than a helpless substitute for crying, but all the same I was relieved to hear it.

An hour or so later Ed took me back to my hotel with an admonition to get a good sleep, but I hardly slept at all that night. I was frightened about my appearance in court the next day. Meeting Tom Wilson's family had given a new reality to the case, to my desire to help, to be a cool and clever expert witness. And my visit had been disturbing in more ways than this. I recalled Paula's intensity when she first told me about this case, her sharp sense of outrage. I understood better now her instinctive feelings, her pained sense of identification. For the first time I was seeing a patient's experience from their point of view alone, and it was, I admit, thoroughly unnerving.

The trial began early that morning. The courtroom was bigger than I thought it would be. It was in an old building, a somber high-ceilinged room filled with tall dark benches. A red-haired man in a gray suit was sitting at a table across the room, and I figured by his steely glance at me that he was the defendant, Dr. Carson. Clara Wilson came into the courtroom and gave me a tentative little nod. She was wearing a navy-blue suit that made her look very young and vulnerable.

"I hope I'm going to be a good witness," I whispered to Ed Baker.

He gave me a reassuring nod, and then the jury came in. Four women and eight men. As I studied their faces my apprehension increased. It seemed to me that they all wore the same kind of closed and guarded expression.

After what seemed an interminable amount of time the judge came in, the court was called to order and the trial began.

The first person called to the stand by Ed Baker was Dr. Randolph, the defendant's partner, a tall, slightly stooped balding man.

Q. Doctor, directing your attention to Saturday, September 21. On that day you were to take over and see the patients of Dr. Carson when he was to be off on the weekend, isn't that true?

A. That's right.

Q. And this included seeing Tom Wilson, isn't that true?

A. That's right.

Q. Would you interpret for us what is said on that slip with reference to Wilson?

A. It gives his room number and his name, of course, and then after this it says: "Post drunk. Broken ribs? URI [upper respiratory infection]."

Q. Doctor, it is true, is it not, that Dr. Carson did not tell you that this man had a possible abdominal injury?

A. I do not recall that he did, no.

Q. Now, Doctor, it is true, isn't it, that the normal and customary practice at Clayton, Arizona, for a physician treating a patient with a suspected abdominal injury, would [be to] notify a doctor who was going to take over the case, is that true?

A. Yes, he would mention that this man has a possible abdominal injury.

Q. Now on Saturday evening, you went to the hospital to see your patients and those of Dr. Carson, is that correct?

A. Yes.

Q. And will you tell us just in narrative form what happened so far as Tom Wilson is concerned.

I glanced around to see how Mrs. Wilson was taking all this. She was sitting very straight, with her chin held high, and though she was very pale her face was composed.

A. Well, I went to the hospital I would say around seven or so, and I started making rounds. I usually start on the fourth floor; and I had about three patients to see there, which I saw. Then I came down to the third floor, to the area that we call three center; and I was standing, starting to look at the charts, when the nurse came running up and said, "Come quick, this patient is very sick," or words to that effect. So I went running down to the room where Mr. Wilson was, and went in and at that time he was obviously in extremis.

Q. What do you mean by extremis?

A. Well, I mean that he was almost dead, and was making a few gasping respirations. I quickly checked him and I could not detect any heartbeat. I did not take his blood pressure. I could not feel any pulse. I examined his abdomen very quickly, and it was somewhat distended and tympanitic.

I hadn't expected Dr. Randolph to give an emotional account of the events, of course, but hearing him describe this young man's unnecessary death in the detached monotone of a tired waiter really outraged me. I glanced at the jury. One woman, about Mrs.

Wilson's age, was frowning; the other eleven faces registered no
more feeling than Dr. Randolph's flat Western voice.

Q. Let me see. I think we need help with "tympanitic."

A. It means that if you percuss over the abdomen . . . you
evoke a note which sounds like tapping a high-pitched drum.
It's a hollow sound. And at this point I started to give him
closed-chest cardiac massage.

Q. How was that done?

A. This is done by getting up on the bed where the patient
is, and using your hands and pressing down on the lower end
of the breast bone at a rate of perhaps sixty a minute. . .; and
we have found that by doing this we squeeze the blood out of
the heart into the circulation; and it is possible, at times, to
resuscitate persons who have had their heart stop beating by
this means, although it is not always successful. We also
started breathing for him by means of the emergency equipment that was on the ward, which is an oxygen tank and mask.
However, it became apparent from the fact that his pupils were
dilated and fixed that there was nothing that we could do; and
after about twenty minutes, I discontinued the attempt to
resuscitate him.

Q. Now, following that, you had some conversations with
Mrs. Wilson that evening?

A. Yes.

Q. And she either right away or at least on that evening
authorized an autopsy, did she not?

A. Yes.

Q. And you are familiar with the results of that autopsy?

A. Yes. I read the report over.

Q. Now, just to sum that up, then, Doctor, it's true, is it
not, that this patient's death was caused by a hemorrhage in
which he bled to death internally?

A. Yes.

By the time the court adjourned at noon, my suit jacket was
clinging to me, thoroughly damp with perspiration. Out in the
corridor, Ed and I stopped for a minute to talk with Clara Wilson.

"It's going to be okay," Ed told her.

"Thank you, both of you," she said, her voice so low I could barely hear her. It was the only thing, that small weak voice, that betrayed what she must be going through.

"Ed's right, you know, not to worry," I told her, though by now I myself was very uncertain about the outcome of the trial. To me the judge and the jurors seemed as unmoved and passive as the defendant's witnesses.

"It's a typical courtroom scene. They always look that way," Ed explained to me at lunch. "You're just not used to it. How about that blueberry pie for dessert?"

But he, as it turned out, had as little appetite as I did, and we just sat over our plates of chicken salad and pie trying to reassure each other that the jury would bring in a verdict for young Mrs. Wilson. Dr. Carson had behaved with such obvious negligence that I couldn't imagine how a jury would be able to ignore it.

"You just never know," Ed said, wiping his glasses with his napkin. "Justice can be a pretty elusive thing sometimes. But if anybody can convince this jury of the real facts, Dick, it's you."

This did not, of course, make me feel any calmer, and when we returned to the court for the afternoon session I remember thinking that no operating room had ever made me feel as tense as that courtroom. Along about midafternoon I was finally called to the stand.

"The plaintiff's attorney calls Richard Chodoff to the stand," a voice called out.

Ed Baker gave me an encouraging nod and I took my first steps toward the witness box, startled at how loud my shoes sounded against the hardwood floors, a sound that was marking the end of my life as a conventional medical man.

"Raise your right hand, please."

My hand shot up of its own volition.

"Place your left hand on the Bible."

I felt the eyes of the twelve jurors focused on me in a single gaze.

"Do you swear to tell the truth, the whole truth, and nothing but the truth, so help you God."

"I do." This was it, and as I uttered those two words I remember feeling that I was making at last a complete commitment to the patient.

Q. Please give the court your full name and address.

A. Richard Joseph Chodoff, 2000 Old West Chester Pike, Havertown, Pennsylvania.

Q. Profession?

A. I'm a doctor of medicine.

Q. You're a practicing surgeon, are you not?

A. Yes.

Q. You're a member of the American Board of Surgery?

A. Yes, and a Fellow of the American College of Surgeons.

Q. Are you a member of any other medical societies?

A. Yes, I am. The American Association for Thoracic Surgery, the Philadelphia Academy of Surgery, the Delaware County Medical Society, the American College of Chest Physicians and the AOA Honorary Medical Society.

Q. Thank you, Doctor. Now, turning to your study of this case, what materials have you had in your possession to study it?

A. I have had the hospital records and depositions of the plaintiff, the defendant and other doctors.

I hardly recognized my own voice, it sounded so loud and deep in that somber courtroom.

Q. Were you part of the group that conducted the study in this green book I'm holding which is called *The Management of Fractures and Soft Tissue Injuries?*

A. For a number of years I was a member of the Regional Committee on Trauma of the College of Surgeons in Philadelphia, yes.

Q. Can you tell us what the purpose of that publication was?

A. To standardize and to improve surgical care in all types of trauma, including trauma to the abdomen.

Q. Doctor, based on your knowledge of this hospital record, the depositions of the defendant, John R. Carson, and the depositions of the other doctors, I will ask you if you have an opinion as to whether or not the care which was given to Tom Wilson by Dr. Carson conformed to the proper standard of practice.

A. Yes, sir, I have an opinion.

Q. And would you state that opinion?

I looked past Ed, out over the courtroom to where the patient's widow sat.

A. I don't believe that this patient was handled according to any of the standards of good surgical care. I think he was inadequately handled.

Q. Would you explain what you feel would have to be done in this particular case as a minimum to meet the adequate proper standard of care?

A. I can tell you what I would do; and I think what I would do is pretty much what any experienced surgeon in the country would do. . . .

I hesitated for a moment, glancing over at the set faces of the jurors, wondering how I could briefly and clearly sum up the necessary action. Ed gave me another encouraging nod, and, taking a deep breath, I plunged into my answer.

. . . The patient would be admitted, examined, a good history taken, the type of injury determined, or the type of force determined which produced the injury . . . if I thought any X rays were needed, I would take them immediately.

I would certainly get a blood count and hematocrit, either one or both; and urinalysis, if possible.

All these things are necessary immediately for one very good reason. You have got to establish a base line for comparison. One blood pressure reading doesn't mean anything. One blood count doesn't mean anything. Perhaps even one X ray doesn't mean anything. But if you get everything at the time you are admitting the patient for observation, you have got something for the future.

Ed gave me a moment to catch my breath and then proceeded along the line of questioning we had more or less rehearsed.

Q. Now, would your opinion be changed at all by the testimony of the defendant doctor that there really were no positive findings of any significance on his examination at 9 A.M. on Saturday morning?

A. No, my opinion would not be changed.

Q. Can you tell us why?

A. In view of the autopsy findings, it is utterly inconceivable to me that this patient had a negative abdomen eight or ten hours before he died. With a torn mesentary, which is bleeding, and with a completely divided small bowel which is spilling intestinal contents into the peritoneal cavity, certainly there would have been some signs.

Q. Can you help us with this spilling contents into the peritoneal cavity?

A. Well, the small intestine leads from the stomach into the large intestine, and then to the rectum; and the contents in the small intestine are liquid; and when it is divided the things spill. To give a homely analogy—if you hooked up a hose in your kitchen to your yard to wash your car, and somebody came along with a knife and cut the hose, you wouldn't get any water to the car; but you would get a lot of water on your kitchen floor; so when this bowel is cut the way it was, the contents just spill into the peritoneal, abdominal cavity.

Q. Doctor, with reference to pain, when the contents spill, as you put it, on the kitchen floor or the abdominal cavity, where would you find the pain?

A. You find pain all over the abdomen.

Q. Thank you, Doctor. Your witness.

This was the moment I had been dreading, the cross-examination by Dr. Carson's lawyer, a Mr. MacIntyre. He was a short stocky fellow with wiry gray hair and a tone so overpolite that it was as aggressive as his stance.

Q. Doctor, I think you told me that this is your first visit to Arizona.

A. Yes, sir.

Q. You have never had any experience in our local hospitals or with our local doctors?

A. No, sir.

Q. Now, back in Philadelphia where you practice, is it a requirement that all orders be written down for nurses?

A. Well, this is a requirement anywhere in the world, sir.

Q. I am asking about Philadelphia.

A. Yes, it is, of course.

Q. You don't know what our practice here in Clayton is, do you?

As he said this, the defense lawyer gave a sidelong glance at the jury that was intended, like his questions, to brand me as an intruder, an interfering outsider, and I hesitated a moment over my answer.

A. No; but I do know that nurses don't carry out orders if they are not written.

Q. Did you have the impression that each time that a nurse took the pulse of Tom Wilson they immediately came out and recorded it on this graphic chart?

A. No, if they do it as they do in most places, the nurse will have what we call a temperature book; and usually the girls go around to all the patients, and record temperatures, pulses, respiration, and write them in the book, and then bring the book out to the nurses' station, and then record them on the chart.

Q. Well, I want to ask you further, then, Doctor, if there is an accepted and standard practice here in the Clayton hospital, that even without a written order the nurse will call a doctor if something unusual or abnormal is going on with a patient, would you say that if this chart is correct, the doctor should have been called?

A. Most certainly.

Q. Doctor, I am getting into something that I am not sure that I am qualified to get into, and you are going to have to help me out here. Whether or not a surgeon goes into an abdomen depends upon the final evaluation that you make of that abdomen, after considering many factors, is that correct?

A. Considering all factors.

Q. Considering all factors. And it's the judgment of the man, the final judgment of the man at the time that determines whether he should or should not?

As I paused to sort out another of Defense Attorney MacIntyre's garbled questions, I could feel the eyes of the twelve jurors on me. I didn't know whether it was a hostile or friendly gaze. The only thing I was sure of was its intensity.

A. Should or should not operate? Yes.

Q. And there are occasions when there is surgery and the patient died, and there was no showing in autopsy of any condition?

A. Are you talking now about traumatic cases, or in general?

Q. Well, let's make it in cases of trauma.

A. I suppose there are. I don't know of any cases in which a person with a negative abdomen and exploration died.

Q. Of course, a very capable man such as you are is not as likely to lose a patient as someone less capable, isn't that correct?

A. This is a very difficult question for me to answer.

Q. Well, don't be bashful.

Mr. MacIntyre turned to share his little private smile with the jury, and I knew he was waiting for me to show myself as a fool. I took a deep breath and, remembering Ed Baker's advice, answered as calmly and objectively as I could.

A. I would say that anybody who has been certified by the Board in surgery is probably capable of handling a situation as well as anyone else. Now, the degree of skill I think comes with experience and years, but I think any Board-certified surgeon could handle this situation.

Q. There are many intangibles that enter into it, his impressions that he gets from the mannerisms of the patient, what he sees, and that sort of thing affects his judgment.

A. I would say not in a situation like this, no.

Q. Wouldn't you say that the physical examination is one of the most important things?

A. Yes, but this is not an intangible. This is very tangible.

Q. Maybe I am misusing the term, then, but the things which he sees and observes are the things that he evaluates?

A. Yes.

Q. And that's of course from the standpoint of the length of time that he has been a doctor and his ability and that sort of thing?

A. The more experience he has, the better he is able to evaluate, I imagine.

Q. Well, the cases that you as a very, very capable surgeon are required to come in and look at are cases where there is already a suspicion that something severe is going on, isn't that true?

A. Well, a patient who has been in an automobile accident, and who has an abdominal injury, is usually seen by a surgeon immediately . . .

Q. Is that back in your country where you practice?

A. Yes, sir.

Q. That could be quite different out here in Arizona.

A. I suppose it could be, but I don't know.

I was dismissed with a shrug for the jury's benefit—a sort of what-is-this-stranger-doing-in-our-town gesture. I glanced over at Clara Wilson. Her face showed the signs of strain and fatigue one usually sees on a woman twice her age. I was afraid to look at the jury. I simply hoped with all my heart that MacIntyre had not succeeded in prejudicing them.

Ed Baker invited me to his mother's house for dinner, but I begged off, telling him that I was exhausted and wanted to get back to the hotel to bathe and go over some notes for the next day. This was true enough, but what I was really looking forward to was talking to Paula, and I didn't even wait to take off my jacket before calling our home number.

"Dick! How was it there today?"

"Hot and sticky."

Over the phone I could hear the intake of breath that preceded her deep laugh. "I was talking about the trial."

"So was I, darling. I don't find it very . . . comfortable."

"I don't think you're supposed to. Only easy things are comfortable—that's a quote. From Dr. Chodoff."

"I'm afraid I recognize it."

"Please be serious and tell me how you are and how things are going."

"I miss you, but I'm fine. And I don't know about the trial—that's the trouble. Definitely I'm the outsider, and how welcome my testimony is I can't tell. It's an unbelievable case. Worse than I thought. The negligence, the utter disregard Wilson was treated with—it's scandalous. As for his young widow, well, it's a heartbreaking situation. I just hope to God I'm doing her some good by being here."

"If any surgeon's testimony can help her, it's yours."

"That's what Baker says."

"Then be grateful you're in a position to do good. What's right and true has to triumph. Besides—I love you."

I smiled across the empty hotel room. "That's a non sequitur."

Paula laughed. "I don't think my loving you could ever be a non sequitur."

Though our conversation helped me to sleep well that night, I woke up to an increased anxiety over Mrs. Wilson and her children. I could not imagine how she would manage to get along if the case was lost. Ed came over to have breakfast with me, and then we returned to the court, where I waited with ill-concealed agitation for him to call me back to the stand.

Q. Would you tell us whether in your opinion the standard of care is the same for patients who have been drinking as for patients who have not?

A. The standards are the same, and we even have to be more careful in a person who has been drinking, as his responses may not be normal. He may not be able to tell you as accurately as a sober person whether he hurts and whether he has got tenderness when you examine him.

Q. In your opinion, would the fact that this patient was intoxicated on admission have anything to do with the failure to diagnose the case?

A. No, sir.

Q. Doctor, have you operated on cases which are similar to the injuries that this man had?

A. Yes, I have.

Q. Do you have any idea how many such operations you have performed?

A. I suppose over the last fifteen or twenty years I have done forty, fifty, sixty, I really don't know; but I have either operated myself or been in charge of a patient like this, of three so far this year, two with identical injuries such as this and one with a lacerated liver.

Q. Are these operations commonly successful?

A. Yes, practically always, unless there are other major associated injuries.

Q. Dr. Chodoff, you are aware that in this case the Clayton Hospital at the time of this incident did not have an intensive-care unit.

A. Yes.

Q. And you are also aware that the Clayton Hospital does not have interns and residents, aren't you?

A. Yes.

Q. In your opinion . . . is the minimum standard of care that you have testified should have been followed altered in any way because of the fact that the hospital doesn't have intensive-care units, doesn't have interns or residents?

A. No, it just makes it a little more difficult for the attending physician; but the standards of care are the same.

Q. Would the increased difficulty to the attending physician be justification for failing to do the things that you have testified should have been done?

I was aware of the jurors imperceptibly leaning forward to hear my answer. Looking over the courtroom to where Clara Wilson sat, I gave a loud firm reply.

A. No, I don't think it would.

Q. And, Doctor, incidentally, is it customary and ordinary in these cases to order the nurses to record changes and observe the patient carefully?

A. In a situation like this where there are no interns or residents, I think one of the most important orders that can be left on a patient's chart, if the attending physician is not in the building during the night, which I assume he was not, is to leave an order for the nurse or whoever is in charge of the floor, the supervisor, to call the physician if there is any change in any way in the patient's condition. In other words, if his pulse goes up, if he complains of abdominal pain, if his blood pressure goes down, if his hematocrit or hemoglobin drops, or if anything unusual happens, you leave an order to be called immediately.

Q. Now, based, then, on your study of the record, of the depositions, based on your experience . . . do you have an opinion as to whether this patient would have survived if the minimum standard of care which you have testified to had in fact been followed in the case?

Mr. MacIntyre: Objection, Your Honor.

The Court: Overruled. You may answer.

A. It is my opinion that if this patient had been operated on the morning of the day following his injury, in view of what was found at autopsy, which were very, very easily correctable injuries, that his chances of walking out of the hospital would have been far greater than ninety percent, I would say pretty close to one hundred percent.

After my testimony I went straight to the airport to catch an afternoon flight back home. The next day a jubilant Ed Baker called me at my office to tell me the jury had brought in a verdict for Mrs. Wilson, the largest verdict in Arizona history.

That night when we sat down to dinner Paula surprised me with a bottle of champagne. "A toast to justice, to Ed Baker and to you, my darling. The rest of the bottle," she said, her green eyes sparkling, "we'll drink to Shakespeare for 'The quality of mercy is not strain'd.'"

3

THE WEEK AFTER I got back from Arizona, Paula and I were invited
to a colleague's silver wedding anniversary party. It was a big happy
event—half the doctors of Philadelphia were there. The food was
superb, the liquor even better, and I, still high on the verdict for
Clara Wilson, was celebrating for everybody.

"Dr. Chodoff, I presume?"

I turned around from the bar to see Daniel Haber, who has been
my good friend since our medical-school days.

"Dan! I was going to call you for lunch. What's your schedule
this week?"

"Heavy, very heavy." He sat down next to me, a dark wiry man
whose shaggy gray mustache and leonine head made him look
rather like Albert Einstein, and whose work in cardiac surgery has
made him worthy of the resemblance. "Michael said you were out
West."

"Did he tell you why?"

Dan nodded and gave me an appraising look. "A gutsy thing to
do, Dick. I don't know how wise, but gutsy, yes."

"It was a horrible affair. Once I reviewed the hospital files there
was no way I could, in good conscience, refuse to be an expert
witness for the plaintiff," I told Dan, and gave him a summary of
Tom Wilson's case.

Several doctor friends had by now joined us, and one of them

49

said to me, "Well, it's a lousy case, sure, but you really ought to have thought twice before interfering."

Inwardly I flinched at his choice of words. "Oh, I thought twice, all right," I assured him, recalling with a grim smile the soul-searching that had led me to this inevitable moment of reprisal.

Dan, meanwhile, was lifting a bristling eyebrow at our colleague. "A lousy case, you call it? That's an understatement. I say it's outrageous. They as good as killed the patient."

"But we're talking about a case out in Arizona, for God's sake," another surgeon protested. "What business was it of Dick's to go butting into something that happened in another state?"

I hesitated before answering. "The same business, I guess, that keeps me at the hospital: a responsibility to the patient, his family— to the medical profession, for that matter."

"Well, the profession has another name for that kind of responsi-bility," said a casual acquaintance, an internist at Mount Sinai Hospital. "They call it treachery." And with that he walked away.

There was an awkward silence, which Dan broke by suggesting another round of drinks. I think he was hoping for another round of conversation as well, but a neurosurgeon friend said, "I've got to admit, Dick, I find it very hard to understand why you'd go all the way to Arizona to testify against another doctor."

"That isn't altogether the way I saw it, Sam. I figured I was going out there to testify for the patient's widow."

"Well, in my books," a newcomer to the group said, "that's unethical behavior."

"Fortunately, we don't keep the same books." I could feel myself getting hot under the collar. "Perhaps it's time we redefine some terms. Why is it ethical to protect a colleague who's guilty of the most flagrant negligence and unethical to pity the injured patient?"

At this point the little South American band hired for the occasion began to serenade the anniversary couple. Paula and Dan's wife, Beatrice, came over to join us, and that ended what I suspected was only the first, and probably mildest, of my social debates in the medical community.

In the months that followed I was asked to review an increasing number of cases. There were very few reputable surgeons in the early 1970s who would admit in public that the medical profession had its occasional offender, that an injured patient has a right to seek redress in the law. So it wasn't surprising that I began getting phone calls from attorneys all over the country who had heard that Dr. Chodoff was a legitimate expert willing to stand up as a witness for the plaintiff.

It was not always an easy thing for me, a man of sixty-three by this time, to continue striking out against tradition. Though committed to following the dictates of my conscience, I still had some shaky moments, distressing times of feeling like an alien in my professional world. And, to a certain degree, in my family, for I did not exactly receive the blessings of my two brothers. Paul, a prominent psychiatrist and author, had a somewhat ambivalent reaction. In general, his sympathies leaned toward the physician. He felt that the times were already too litigious, though he did agree with me that suit is justified when gross negligence has occurred.

My youngest brother, Pete, a well-known anesthesiologist and author, was violently opposed to my stand, and we got into some terrible arguments. The word "malpractice" was anathema to Pete, as to most doctors, and he held angrily to the dogma that a doctor is entitled to a "mistake" and should be forgiven even if it costs the patient life or limb.

Though I argued with him, I understood and could sympathize with, up to a point, his prejudices, which in part stemmed from a most unhappy incident that took place early in his career. Pete had been the anesthesiologist in charge of a patient who was having his gall bladder removed. The surgeon got into trouble and called for a unit of blood to be given. The blood was delivered, and, as required, Pete checked it for the name, unit number and room number. All seemed to be in order, so he gave the blood. Unfortunately, it turned out that there were two patients with the same name on the same floor. The laboratory sent the other patient's blood type to the operating room with the wrong room number on the bottle. Pete's patient developed a massive transfusion reaction and, after a series of hematologic and surgical complications, died. A malpractice suit was brought against the hospital, the surgeon and Pete, who was truly an innocent bystander in this tragedy. Though he had to spend two highly uncomfortable weeks in court as a defendant, he was found innocent of any negligence. It was a traumatic experience and had, I knew, a great deal to do with his present attitude.

But that attitude was, of course, the prevailing one in the medical profession. Mine was an unpopular cause and I was frankly grateful for the encouragement and support I got from those closest to me. My son Bill, a pediatrician and, like my father, the most compassionate of doctors, gave me his wholehearted approval. Virginia Maxwell, my secretary for more than a dozen years, continued to be a devoted, loyal friend, generously extending her kindness to those injured patients who sometimes visited my office.

And as for Paula, well, I had never before been able to share so much of my life with anybody. Our mutual concern for the patient plaintiff was becoming an integral part of our life together. More often than not, when we lingered over dinner, or went to sit by the fire in my study, it was to continue a conversation about some new case, occasionally a medical file that Paula had asked me to evaluate.

I should emphasize that ninety percent of the records I reviewed involved surgical complications that had nothing to do with malpractice. But there was always that one-out-of-ten file in which negligence had occurred either in the treatment or in the general standard of care. Or in the diagnosis. One such case in which I became involved had to do with the consistent failure of a radiologist to make an obvious diagnosis of lung cancer.

The purpose of periodic chest X rays in patients without symptoms is to detect this deadly disease as early as possible. Every textbook will confirm the fact that the earlier the diagnosis of lung cancer, and treatment, the better the chance for cure. Yet in the case of Henry Neuman, a forty-five-year-old Connecticut man, an early and roentgenologically obvious tumor was overlooked each year for three years, incredible negligence that denied him the possibility of curative pulmonary resection and, ultimately, took his life.

At the time of his first X ray in 1968 Mr. Neuman was a heavy smoker but an apparently healthy man. His was, by all standards, a happy and successful life. A well-paid executive of a large corporation, he had a comfortable home in the suburbs, an attractive wife and two teenaged sons.

One of the benefits that Mr. Neuman's company gave its executives was a complete annual physical examination which included blood tests, cardiograms and chest X rays. Each year he received a clean bill of health, including a notation that his chest X ray showed no abnormalities.

Henry Neuman's ambition was to one day run his own advertising firm, and in January of 1971 he and his wife, Beth, decided that the future looked bright enough to take a few risks. By using most of their savings and re-mortgaging their home, Henry was able to quit his job and start his own agency.

That March, a year from the date of his last physical examination as a company employee, he arranged for a checkup with Dr. J. J. Saunders, an old family friend who practiced in New Haven. The chest X ray that Dr. Saunders took revealed a large, abnormal shadow in the upper lobe of the right lung, and Henry was hospitalized at once. Complete studies, including bronchoscopy and biopsy, indicated a cancer in the right upper lobe, and an operation was promptly scheduled. Despite the fact that several of the lymph nodes in the root of the lobe were enlarged, the surgeon made an attempt to remove it. The pathologic report showed the usual type of lung cancer, but, unfortunately, all of the enlarged nodes were found to contain cancer.

The Neuman family's life underwent a sudden and drastic change. The new business was abandoned at a great loss, and what money was salvaged went into medical bills. Henry was in and out of the hospital, first on a course of X-ray therapy and then for intensive chemotherapy. He suffered all the side effects of his treatments: nausea, loss of appetite, loss of hair, and anemia. Within a few months he began to complain of increasing fatigability and shortness of breath. Spread of the cancer to his bones, liver and other organs was soon confirmed, and Henry Neuman lived out his few remaining months confined to a bed with the most intense pain.

Dr. Saunders, an alert and ethical physician, was naturally curious about the annual chest X rays taken while Henry was in his former company's employ. He requested the films for 1968, 1969 and 1970 and discovered, unsurprisingly, that they were not "normal" as the radiologist had claimed. He then advised his friend's widow that, in his opinion, legal action was called for.

Shortly thereafter, I received a call from Beth Neuman's attorney, who explained the entire family situation to me and asked if I would review the case. I agreed to do so, and within several days the medical records and films of the three annual examinations taken prior to Henry Neuman's resignation arrived at my office.

I remember as clearly as if it had been last week the morning I took those X rays to the view boxes in our X-ray department. They were hung in order, and one of the technicians who happened to be walking by stopped, pointed to the first film and said, "That area certainly looks suspicious, doesn't it?"

Indeed it did, and if this was obvious enough to be commented on by a passing technician, how, then, could it have been missed for three consecutive years by a qualified radiologist? The most likely explanation was the most damning—that he had simply never looked at them.

Reviewing the films with a radiologist friend, I found that the 1968 X ray showed an abnormal density about one and a half centimeters in diameter in the right upper lobe. Such a finding, especially in a middle-aged man, a heavy smoker, demanded two actions. First, comparison with any previous chest films to see if the abnormality had been present before. Second, assuming that it was a new finding, a repeat X-ray in about a month was mandatory, since one could reasonably expect the area to have cleared if it were due to inflammation. Had it persisted on the repeat film, then investigation should have been undertaken to determine whether this abnormality represented a cancer of the lung. Yet nothing was done, nor was Mr. Neuman warned of anything wrong.

The chest X rays taken in 1969 and 1970 showed the same area of abnormality, except that it was denser and had increased in size. As these films did not yet show any involvement of the lymph nodes, it was reasonable to assume that curative surgery might have been achieved in 1968. No doubt remained in my mind that the radiologist was guilty of the grossest carelessness, and I told the plaintiff's attorney that in my opinion this negligence had deprived Henry Neuman of any chance of survival.

The case was completely indefensible, and I was not surprised to learn that after suit was brought against the radiologist his malpractice-insurance company settled with the Neuman family out of court.

I was still naïve enough to consider the Neuman case a monstrous rarity, yet not three months later Paula was engaged as the medical-legal consultant on a similarly shocking case. This time it was a middle-aged woman whose cancer of the breast went undiagnosed for over two years despite her periodic visits to a well-known gynecologist.

I first heard the story when I came home from the hospital one night to find Paula still at work.

"You're late. Am I glad to see you!" she said.

"What's wrong?"

Her face, unusually strained with fatigue, relaxed into a smile as she came over to kiss me. She hesitated. "I wasn't going to bother you with it tonight—sure you don't mind shop talk?"

"Since when? I'll mix us a nightcap and you can tell me what's got you upset."

"So much for what I fondly think of as my poker face," Paula said, sitting down again at her desk, her hair a shining, almost glossy black under the lamp. "Well, you're right—I am upset. There's a medical file I want you to review, Dick. I know you've got a lot of surgery scheduled this week, but, if it's possible, I'd really like to have your opinion on this case."

"Can you fill me in a little?"

"It's a client of Mel Osborne's," Paula said, naming an attorney friend in Trenton, New Jersey. "A woman named Frascotti. Maria Frascotti. Widowed, fifty years old, a hairdresser. Used to be, anyway. Well, about three years ago she discovered a small lump in her breast, and she did just what all those medical warnings say to do—went to her gynecologist and explained exactly where and how she found it. And did she get the good doctor's sympathetic attention? No. The arrogant SOB told her he didn't need a patient to tell him how to handle an examination, and he dismissed the whole thing. Repeatedly."

"And she didn't go for another opinion?"

Paula shook her head. "Not for two years. He continued to tell her in later examinations that nothing was wrong, and she believed him. You know the type, they have a kind of . . . reverence for doctors. Finally her sister got her to a surgeon, who did a radical mastectomy almost immediately, but by this time, of course, the cancer had spread to the axillary nodes. So she had to have postoperative radiation, and that left her with such bad edema that she can't use her arm anymore and had to quit her job. Some bedtime story, right?" Paula said bitterly. "She's a very nice lady, too, this Maria Frascotti. Mel said she was reluctant to bring suit. Didn't think she had any rights, you know. After all, he was the Doctor, the great authority figure. In fact, it was the sister's husband who finally took charge and brought her to see Mel."

I sighed, tired suddenly, and sad. "Tomorrow's busy, but I'll get a start on the case somehow."

Like Paula, I was profoundly disturbed by what I read in Maria Frascotti's medical files, and I arranged for her to come to Philadelphia to see me the following week.

"Pleased to meet you, Dr. Chodoff," she said as Mrs. Maxwell showed her into the office. "I hope I'm pronouncing your name right. In Italy they say the *Ch* different, like Chianti." She was a large, round-faced woman whose sparkling dark eyes and animated manner gave her a youthful air. "Of course, I've been in America since I was a kid, but some things stay with you no matter."

"Yours is a very lovely homeland," I told her. "Please sit down, Mrs. Frascotti. Will you be comfortable enough?"

"Me? Oh, sure, absolutely." But for all her cheerful manner she could no more hide the discomfort of her swollen arm than she could the small lines of pain etched around her mouth.

"Where in Italy were you born?"

"Naples, both me and my husband. He's gone now, God rest his soul."

"It's a beautiful city. My wife, Paula, and I had the good fortune to visit it on our honeymoon several years ago."

Mrs. Frascotti smiled broadly. "If it was your honeymoon you must've taken the boat over to Capri, too, am I right?" And with this casual conversation, and the cup of tea Mrs. Maxwell thoughtfully provided, she relaxed and we began to discuss her case.

"I was always reading articles about breast cancer," she told me. "How important it was to discover it early. I was a hairdresser, you know, and we got these women's magazines at the beauty shop all the time. Anyway, I learned how to do the self-examinations, and I was really careful to keep a good check on myself. Then, sure enough, about three years ago I felt this lump up on the outer part of my right breast. It was small like a little knot and it wasn't all that easy to find. I mean I could only feel it if I was lying down with my arm up over my head and my body sort of tilted."

"That's when you saw the general practitioner?"

"Dr. Rudy, right. He was our family doctor. My sister and her kids went to him, too."

"And was he able to locate the lump?"

Mrs. Frascotti nodded, shifting the weight of her swollen useless arm. "Sure. I lay down the same way and he felt it, too. He told me it was about the size of a small coin, and I should go see a surgeon. But I already had this appointment fixed for my usual checkup with my gynecologist. So Dr. Rudy said, 'Okay, when you see Dr. Dunhill next week you tell him about this and then follow his recommendations.' "

For the first time a look of sad bewilderment came over Maria Frascotti's face. "You know, Dr. Chodoff, I still can't believe it could have happened the way it did. I said to Dr. Dunhill, 'I found a lump in my right breast; Dr. Rudy also found it, but you can only feel it when I'm lying flat on my back, a little tilted, with my arm up.' " Mrs. Frascotti paused again. "The way Dr. Dunhill looked at me. Like I'd said something nasty, insulted him. 'Mrs. Frascotti, I've examined thousands of female breasts,' he said in this very cold voice. 'No patient has to tell me how it's done.' "

"Did he examine you then?"

"Yes, but not in the right position." She blushed. "I mean not in the position where I told him he'd be able to feel the lump. It was like he purposefully avoided it. Then he said there wasn't any lump, that I was probably imagining things because of all the cancer publicity."

"He didn't suggest getting a surgeon's opinion or having mammograms done?"

"No, he said I was okay and to come back in six months." Mrs. Frascotti shifted her arm again. "To tell you the truth, it's this thing here that's driving me crazy. All this pain and swelling from the radiation. That's why I had to stop work. You can get used to having your breast gone, I guess, but the way my arm hurts sometimes I think I can't take it anymore."

"I'm sorry, Mrs. Frascotti. I know how uncomfortable you must be and I won't keep you any longer. There's just one last question: During the following year and a half that you visited Dr. Dunhill, did you continue to be conscious of a mass in your right breast?"

She looked at me with her dark eyes wide and grave. "Oh, yes, sure I was. But Dr. Dunhill always said everything was all right." And her earnest explanation, which I thought about after she left, made me think of the patients of a generation ago, those loving Italians who had come to my father's office. I realized that, like them, her faith and devotion was such that she'd no more have questioned her doctor's opinion than her priest's.

An early diagnosis of breast cancer is the most important weapon we have against this killer disease. Early prompt action can sometimes double a woman's chance for long term survival. By the time Maria Frascotti went to a surgeon, her "small" lump had developed into a large, hard mass. The pathology report revealed that the cancer was fortunately of a fairly low-grade malignancy. However, it was extensive and involved several of her axillary lymph nodes.

Since it was this surgeon's custom to give postoperative radiation treatment to all patients with involved axillary nodes, Mrs. Frascotti was subjected to the prescribed series of X-ray treatments. One of the possible consequences of post-mastectomy radiation is a swelling in the arm, and this Mrs. Frascotti suffered to a severe and disabling degree. Had she been operated upon two years earlier, when she herself discovered the lump in her breast, it is highly unlikely that the cancer would have spread to her axillary nodes.

It is still incomprehensible to me that Dr. Dunhill, a well-trained gynecologist, could have failed repeatedly to detect Mrs. Frascotti's tumor. It is not uncommon for a physician to have trouble locating a lump his patient discovered in her breast. Nor is it unusual, perhaps, for him to feel a measure of embarrassment at having to ask the patient to demonstrate the mass for him. But ask he does, or he should not be allowed to call himself a physician.

That Dr. Dunhill could have dismissed Mrs. Frascotti's findings out of pique, that he did not suggest a further investigation, that he should have allowed his ego to come before her well-being, represented to me a negligence of inhuman proportion. This I reported to Paula and to Mrs. Frascotti's lawyer, Mel Osborne, informing them both that I would be glad, under the circumstances, to stand as the expert witness for the plaintiff.

A malpractice suit generally takes anywhere from twelve months to five years to come to trial. Mrs. Frascotti's case was one of the exceptions, and after only six months I was on my way to Trenton, New Jersey, to appear in court for the second time. I was prepared for almost anything, I think, but a biased judge.

Early diagnosis and treatment of breast cancer is a fact accepted by ninety-nine percent of the medical profession as a means to increase survival rates. A few doctors have tried to refute this. To counter their unwarranted statements, the American Cancer Society has published a pamphlet citing the evidence that early diagnosis is vital. The introductory paragraph of this pamphlet states that some men have argued that the ultimate prognosis of breast cancer does not depend on its early diagnosis. The rest of the document then goes on to thoroughly disprove this argument.

In court the defense attorney read the first paragraph of the pamphlet to me and asked, "Doctor, do you agree with this statement?" When I tried to explain that the paragraph was taken out of context, and was in no way indicative of the rest of the pamphlet, I was sternly admonished by the judge to answer yes or no. My request that the entire pamphlet be read was refused and the judge warned me not to interfere with the course of the trial. I insisted that a yes or no answer was impossible. The trial continued in this way, with increasingly prejudicial statements from the bench. When all testimony had been concluded, the judge rendered his charge to the jury. Needless to say, it virtually directed the jury to return a not-guilty verdict.

While the jury deliberated, the defense attorney settled the case—for a ridiculously small sum. Dr. Dunhill's pride had been vindicated, Anna Frascotti was left with a shortened life expectancy and a painful, useless arm, and a travesty had been made of justice.

About a week after the trial I ran into my friend Daniel Haber as I was leaving the hospital.

"I've been looking for you, Dick. Do you have time for a coffee?"

"Sure. In the lounge?"

"I'd rather go over to Nick's if you're not in a rush." He had a slightly perplexed look, his bushy eyebrows making a straight line across his brow that with Dan means worry.

We walked over to the little coffee shop across the street from the hospital.

"So what's on your mind?" I asked once we were installed in a booth.

"Oh, one thing and another. I've been thinking a lot about the old days—as the saying goes. You remember the gin we used to make at medical school?"

"Who forgets poison?"

"I, for one. I was trying to remember the recipe. Alcohol, glycerine, oil of anise, right? What have I left out?"

"Juniper berry. Now why don't you tell me what's really on your mind."

Dan tugged at his mustache, a gesture that always precedes his reluctant seriousness. "Okay. I'm worried about you. There's a lot of talk going around, Dick. Nobody can figure out what the hell you're up to. That case in Arizona, well, okay, you went out there and you testified. But, good Lord, man, even I never thought you'd do it again."

"I didn't plan to, you know," I said, trying to sort it out as much for myself as for him. "It's nothing I've planned. But there's nobody willing to stick his neck out for the plaintiff. Not a legitimate expert anyway, you know that."

"Exactly. So why you?"

I shrugged. "Why not?"

"Oh, come on. You know damn well why not. Have you stopped to think what's going to happen to your practice? Some of your colleagues are getting very upset, Dick."

"Doesn't surprise me in the least. I was in that rarefied atmosphere not so long ago, remember? I know the party line: We must protect our own; all the years of study and preparation—can't let a colleague risk losing everything over one mistake . . ."

"Aren't you being a little unfair?" Dan interrupted, "Basically that's all kind of true, after all."

"Ah, but only kind of. They're sophistic, those arguments. For one thing, a mistake, as you know, isn't always a mistake. Like this breast cancer case."

Dan gave me a long, oddly reflective look. "So what are you trying to say?"

"I'm not *trying* to say anything. I'm damn well saying it. I won't buy that way of thinking anymore. It seems to me that it's the patient who does the losing. Even if he wins a lousy case, he's already lost—a limb, a life, somebody he loves. And we're told to confine our worry to the doctor? He gets off pretty easy, don't you think? Look at that gynecologist Dunhill. His insurance rates will go up, but that's the only consequence he'll pay. Is the AMA or the state licensing board going after him? Certainly not. No question of his losing his license. He wasn't even officially reprimanded."

"I think that was a rotten case, Dick, you know that. But you'll admit somebody like Dunhill represents only a small minority of the medical profession."

"Very small, thank God. Most of the cases I've been sent to review have nothing to do with malpractice, nothing at all, and I send them right back. They're little two-hundred-dollar nuisance suits from unscrupulous lawyers."

Dan nodded. "Spare me the details, I know already. It happened to me once when a patient sneezed twice postoperatively."

I laughed. "I've had a couple of those myself. What surgeon

who's been in practice over thirty years hasn't? But I'll tell you something, Danny boy, had I ever been sued in a case in which I knew I'd been guilty of malpractice, I bloody well would have insisted that the insurance company settle the case. I wouldn't sit up in my ivory tower and wait for my colleagues to gather around and rescue me."

Dan sighed. "So we're back to that."

"Well, that's the issue here, isn't it? Because one out of every ten cases I'm sent to review *is* malpractice, *is* negligence, *is* in fact a shocking catastrophe. What am I suppose to do? Keep my mouth shut and let some poor patient or his family go hang in order to protect a doctor's reputation?"

Dan didn't answer. He ordered us more coffee, put too much sugar in his, and then said, "Don't misunderstand me. I admire what you're doing. If I had the guts I might do it myself. But I'm not a crusader. What I don't understand is why suddenly you're one. We saw plenty of things go wrong when we were interns. You never said anything then."

"Sure, we used to follow our chief around and if he fumbled we'd think, well, even a doctor's allowed to make a mistake. But, Dan, when it was plain carelessness I cringed, didn't you?"

"Yes, of course. Remember old Belmont? His patients were hardly getting the best care, but he was the chief. Who was I to say anything? I was just a resident, so I told myself when I had my own practice I'd do better. I suppose that's my point. Maybe we can only be concerned with what we do ourselves. How we handle our own patients. I sympathize with what you're doing, Dick, but I'm afraid it's only going to cause great trouble for you. You're a Don Quixote fighting windmills, my friend, you're not going to bring justice to the world."

"That's hardly my ambition," I replied.

Dan grinned. "I'm not so sure."

It would be a lie to pretend I was untroubled by this talk. My colleagues getting angry didn't bother me—that was hardly news. What did disturb me, however, what made me acutely uncomfortable, was the notion of myself turned into a crusading knight on a white charger. Once more I found myself floundering between past and present loyalties. But this time it was only a brief, passing disturbance. I had come a long way from my establishment days, too great a distance to be even tempted to go back.

This realization was confirmed, once and for all, when shortly after my conversation with Dan I received a call from a lawyer in Ohio asking me to review the file of a woman who had died of a ruptured appendix. It did not take long to establish the fact that this was a case of inexcusable surgical negligence. The autopsy showed a gangrenous ruptured appendix, massive peritonitis and an abdomen filled with pus. The patient had suffered all the classical symptoms of "acute appendicitis," yet the care she received was so below standard that this simple diagnosis was never made.

Along with the hospital records the lawyer sent a statement written by the patient's husband. This personal documentation of malpractice, this agonized lament put a final end to whatever lingering doubts I may still have had about testifying for the plaintiff. The statement appears below exactly as I first read it.

STATEMENT OF FRANK CRAVEN REGARDING THE
SURROUNDINGS OF MY WIFE, SUSAN'S, DEATH

I work for the Bell Telephone Company in Morgantown, Ohio, and also operate a flying school at Morgantown County Airport in my spare time. I worked overtime on the night of January 16, 1970, until 11:50 P.M. Upon arriving home around 12:04 my wife Susan met me at the door stating she has some stomach pains since 7 o'clock that evening. I asked her what she had for supper and she said tuna fish. I thought it might be the salad that upset her stomach and asked her to take a couple of aspirins and if that didn't help we would go to the hospital. We both went to bed around 12:30. Early Saturday morning around 4:30 she awoke me stating her stomach pains were quite severe so I called the hospital and told them I was bringing her down which I did shortly afterwards. Upon arriving at the emergency room, the nurse in attendance had her lie down on the bed while she called the doctor on duty whom I believe was Dr. Daley. About twenty minutes later he arrived on the scene and proceeded to ask her questions about her pain and if she had diarrhoea, which she said yes. He asked her when they started and she told him around 7:00 o'clock the previous evening. He asked her what she had for dinner and she told him tuna fish salad. He made the remark that the tuna these days was something else. After about ten more minutes or so, he said that she had a stomach infection. They did not take a blood count at this time and as far as I can remember I did not see them take her temperature either. He said he would give me a prescription to get filled. I told him that it was too early in the morning, I believe around 6:00 at that time, to get a prescription filled, and could he give me something for her then. He put some or rather I believe he had one of the nurses put some liquid type medicine in a bottle and gave it to me. It looked like Pepto Bismol but I could not say for sure. I took her home and she still seemed in severe pain. She usually smiles but this time I could not get her to smile at all. I called my daughter to come down if she could and stay with her as I had a few students scheduled to fly that day. I came home around 5:00 o'clock, Jan. 17, and fixed her some soft boiled eggs which she tried to eat but not too successfully. She kept complaining about her severe pains and when I tried to touch her stomach she would push my hand away in pain. I fell asleep about 11:00 Saturday night and woke up around 7:00. I asked her how she felt and she just nodded her head in a negative sort of way. I fixed her some soft boiled eggs again, and toast, but she ate very little. My daughter Veronica was coming down around 10:00 Sunday morning Jan. 18 to be with my wife as I had a few students scheduled to fly Sunday morning. About 11:30 in the morning my phone at the airport office was ringing and when I answered it my son told me that my daughter Veronica was going to take my wife back down to the hospital due to the severity of the stomach pains. I said I would come right down. I got to the hospital about 12:15 and saw my wife and daughter sitting in the waiting room. I asked her what were they doing there and my daughter replied that they were waiting to be called into the emergency room. I went into the emergency room and the nurses there just seemed to be doing nothing, so I got my dander up and told them what was my wife doing out there with all that pain waiting for them to make up their minds to see her. They told me to bring her right in and we did. They put her on the bed in the emergency room and called for the doctor on duty again. This time they took a blood count. After lying there for about fifteen minutes Dr. Howell appeared on the scene. I explained to him about her condition and thought maybe she might be having a kidney stone attack as she had one previously about a year ago and Dr. Hogan and Dr. Riley took care of her then as Dr. Howell was on vacation. He, Dr. Howell, had the nurse help my wife into the bathroom for a urinalysis specimen. She was in so much pain then she could hardly get out of bed and had to go back in the bathroom twice before she could get her kidneys to function enough for a specimen. During this period of time the blood count came back and I overheard the nurse say to someone behind the drawn curtain that you better look at this or something to that effect. I became very concerned then. A few minutes later Dr. Howell told me that he was giving me three prescriptions to get filled for her. I told him that I did not want any prescriptions, that I wanted her admitted for a few days for observation to see what was the matter with her. He stepped out momentarily and I believe made a phone call and came back and told me that there were no beds available and that she would have to be put in the hall but due to all the inconvenience of the traffic in the hall, he said to me, you wouldn't want her out in the hall with all that confusion etc. and that the prescriptions and medications would take care of her, that she had an infection in her stomach and that he was positive that the medicine would take care of her. I again insisted that I had her down there on Saturday morning Jan. 17 and didn't want to take her home again. He assured me that she would be alright and for me to check with him, I believe he said, Monday or Tuesday, to bring her down to his office. I thought that at this time he knew what he was talking about, so I took my wife out of the hospital and to my car. She could hardly walk to the car. I believe the time of day was around 1:00 Sunday afternoon but I am not positive of the time. My daughter stopped off at the Drugstore at 15th Street and 7th Avenue in Morgantown, and picked up the three prescriptions. When she brought them home I noticed that all three read, one after every meal. I could not figure out when she would get them as she could not keep any food down and didn't want to eat. So we gave them to her periodically at our meal time. She slept a little Sunday evening Jan. 18. I arranged for my daughter to come down around 9:00 in the mornings while I went to work. Before I left for work Monday morning Jan. 19, I wanted to fix her breakfast but she refused it. I called my daughter around noon time the same day to see how she was doing and my daughter replied about the same, and that she couldn't keep any food down. I got home around five o'clock Monday evening and sat down along beside her and talked a little about our proposed trip to Honolulu for our vacation. She didn't seem at all attentive and complained about her stomach aching. I got out our Doctor book and started reading to her different things I thought it might be and when I came to the part about ruptured appendix and peritonitis I said I don't think you have that, honey, or the doctor would have known at the hospital but I remarked, it could be that. She seemed kind of dazed that evening and I asked her to smile but I could not get her to smile at all. The next morning, Tuesday, Jan. 20, I got up and she did not want any breakfast and I told her Veronica would fix her some when she got there at nine. My son, Will, was home all this time as he was recuperating from a sore throat. I phoned my daughter around 10:30 that same morning to see how Susan was doing and she told me not so good, dad. I was then really scared that something was not right so I called Dr. Howell's office right away. He was not in and his nurse asked if I wanted to leave a message. I told her yes, that I wanted my wife admitted to the hospital right away and I told her I didn't care if they had to put my wife in the boiler room, that I wanted her there and left in the hospital until they found out what was wrong. She said Dr. Howell would be calling in and she would give him the message. About 12:30 she called me and said they were admitting my wife to the hospital. My daughter called about thirty minutes later saying they admitted her and had her in a bed in the hall. I was happy she was finally in there where she could get the right attention, I thought. At the same time I told my boss, Mr. Braden, "They finally admitted my wife in the hospital even though it's in the hallway." That evening I came down to the hospital around 6:45 and my daughter was with her. She, my wife, apologized to me for causing me so much trouble and it broke my heart to hear her talk like that, and I said, "Honey, don't worry about a thing, we have hospitalization and everything is going to be alright." She even managed a slight smile for me. I left the hospital around 8:30 and Veronica, my daughter, told me they were going to take X-rays and examine her the next morning on Wednesday, Jan. 21. My daughter told me the next day when I called her at the hospital, or rather when she called me from the hospital, that they took X-rays of mom and put her under a sedative around 10:30 and Dr. Howell and Dr. Maxwell examined her probably in the operating room but I don't know where. My daughter told me when they brought my wife back down that my wife asked her if they operated on her because of the intense pain she had in her stomach. My daughter said she told her no, only an examination and that they were going to put her on medication that evening at 6:00 P.M. My daughter told me the doctors told her that my wife had an infection in the pelvic area and in the urinary tract. She also told me that they would be able to get her a private room that same afternoon. I came down to the hospital that evening, Wednesday, Jan. 21, around 6:30 and sat with her. She looked terrible, but I thought it was the medicine they gave her. She was cold and clammy and all sweaty and I noticed around her throat her heart beat was awfully fast. Around 8:00 she asked one of the nurses if she had something for the pain and the nurse remarked in so many words, that if there was something for the pain in her schedule from the doctor she would give it to her, but there wasn't. I started to take a face cloth and kept rinsing it out with cold water in the bathroom for her forehead as she seemed awfully warm. She told me she wanted the pan as she had to throw up. I rang the buzzer for the nurse but she didn't come so I held the pan under her mouth and she tried pitifully to bring up whatever was bothering her stomach but only saliva seemed to come out. About fifteen minutes after I buzzed for the nurse she walked in and I told her she was trying to throw up. The nurse said to me, "Oh, she is trying to throw up. Okay." And she walked away. I felt she must be some kind of a goon to treat my wife like that. My wife then motioned for some water and she drank a little out through the straw in the glass. By this time her eyes began to look like she was in an hypnotic trance but all the time I thought it was the medicine they must have given her. About 8:50 she asked me if they were going to give her something to sleep so I walked out this time and asked one of the nurses on duty if she was to have something for sleep and the nurse replied yes. I believe she came in about the time I was getting ready to leave, around 9:00. I went home thinking about her and kind of worried but again I felt that the doctors knew what they were doing. Around 4:30 in the morning of Jan. 22 the phone rang. I answered it and the call was as follows: "Mr. Craven?" "Yes," I replied. "This is the hospital supervisor, you'd better come right down." "What's the matter?" I asked. "I don't know," she replied. I got dressed in three or four minutes and went through every stop sign and red light in town to get to her. When I arrived the nurse in the hall outside my wife's room stopped me and said, "Mr. Craven, your wife is dead." I couldn't believe it and must have went into immediate shock. I rushed into her room and held her in my arms crying and begging her not to leave me and told the nurses to do something, but they said she was dead. I wanted to die desperately with her. Sometime in the ensuing few minutes Dr. Howell appeared on the scene. I screamed at him: "What did you do to my wife?" He replied that he didn't know what caused her death and that they would have to do an autopsy to find out. The nurses wanted me to leave my wife then and I told them all to get the hell out of that room and leave me with my wife, and that did they have another patient that needed the room so bad that they couldn't wait for her body to get cold. They left me with my wife for I believe an hour and then the nurse came back in and asked me to sign the autopsy form which I did. They or she told me I should leave as they wanted to start on it right away. I said I wanted to come right back as soon as it was over but when I left the hospital they never called me at all. My daughter took me to Sullivan's funeral home to arrange for the burial and over to Morgantown Memorial Cemetery for the lot. The funeral was on Saturday Jan. 24. I wanted it on Sunday but they don't hold funerals on Sunday they told me at Morgan Memorial. The following week I don't recall which day exactly, I called Dr. Howell and asked him what had happened to my wife. He told me that he wasn't sure, that they had a few more tests to take but he thought it was a ruptured appendix. I flew into a rage and told him it better not appear that way on the death certificate or he would have a lot of explaining to do. He remarked kind of sarcastically that he didn't perform the autopsy and whatever was on it was it. A few days later he called me and said that he would like to get together with me and himself and Dr. Maxwell and go over her case with me. I don't recall the exact day but it was the week of February first I believe. It could have been February 2. It was around 2:00 in the afternoon and I had just come back to work and he wanted me to come to a meeting at 4:00 which I couldn't do and I told him it was too short a notice. He said he would be glad to set up a meeting anytime. I then told him I wanted a copy of the autopsy report and he said what for, I couldn't read it anyway. I said maybe if I can't I'll find an attorney who could. He didn't seem to like that but I can't recall what he said. I called Dr. Maxwell a few days later, I believe, and asked him for the autopsy report. He said if I would stop by he would give me a copy but he would be leaving his office at 4:00 and I couldn't make it until 5:00 and he said he'd be leaving for two weeks vacation and to call Howell for a copy. I decided then to get a hold of a friend of mine, Mr. Tom Patterson, Attorney, who was in the same reserve outfit with me. He said his associate, Mr. Dorman, was out of town and to call him in about ten days. I called him back about a week later and he said that Dorman and Dr. Maxwell were friends and referred me to Mr. Hoffman. I arranged a meeting with Mr. Hoffman. In the meantime, on February 17 I believe, Dr. Howell called me and asked if I could come down to a meeting with him and Dr. Maxwell on February 19 at 8:30 P.M. which I agreed to do. I brought along my son Will. Dr. Howell proceeded to sit there at his desk writing and I said, "Well, you called this meeting." He began to explain about the position of my wife's appendix. After he got through I said, "You are telling me nothing." I asked him why he sent my wife home with those stupid prescriptions, why he let her die and why didn't they take a blood count the first time. He explained that blood counts don't always show infections etc. etc. I then asked Dr. Maxwell point blank how much time he had spent examining her and he couldn't tell me whether it was five minutes or thirty minutes. I said, "If that had been your wife lying there, would you have operated?" He said that he couldn't say. I accused him and Dr. Howell point blank of letting my wife die, and of being criminally negligent and that malpractice took place in their diagnosis of my wife's illness. He tried to explain how these things happen sometimes but his explanations and Dr. Howell's were terribly weak. I said maybe a $500,000 lawsuit would open their mouths and tell me why they didn't operate on her when it was obvious something was seriously wrong. Dr. Maxwell said that he didn't believe she was that sick. When I explained to him her condition when I saw her Wednesday evening January 21 he looked at Dr. Howell and said that he didn't think she was in that kind of shape or some sort of the same line of conversation. Dr. Maxwell then asked me what it was they could do for me. I told them both that I wanted some answers and that their explanations were the worst I ever heard as to what caused her death. I then asked Dr. Howell again for a copy of the autopsy report and he refused it. Dr. Maxwell said to him: "I think Mr. Craven has a right to see it." Still they never got it out for me to see. Howell got a phone call shortly thereafter and I got tired of waiting in his office while he talked about something personal over the phone so I got up to leave and he immediately hung up his phone and came back into the office. Dr. Maxwell asked me what my intentions were and I told him I was going to see my attorney. He said he didn't know what to do as this was the first time anything like this had happened to him. I told him it was my first also, and that his attorney would know what to do, and I left. Dr. Howell proffered me his hand but I refused to accept the handshake. In the few days following I tried to find out from Mrs. Warren, the head nurse at Morgantown Medical Center, the circumstances surrounding my wife's death the morning she died. She advised me to call back in a few hours and she would have the information. When I called back she told me she was sorry but that I would have to talk to the Executive Director. He told me that he could not give me the information since he heard I was taking legal action and referred me to their insurance company in Pittsburgh if I wanted any information.

Mrs. Craven's completely preventable death struck me as a horror story of ignorance and ineptitude. I telephoned the plaintiff's lawyer and told him that in my opinion her death was directly attributable to the outrageous departures from the accepted standards of care by both Dr. Howell and Dr. Maxwell.

After I submitted my report condemning, point by point, the blatant negligence of these two so-called physicians, the insurance company decided against letting the case come to trial. Settlement was made out of court, but no amount of money could compensate Frank Craven for the loss he had suffered.

4

THOUGH MY CONCERN with medical malpractice, and my involvement, were growing steadily deeper, in retrospect this was a peaceful time. So far only one doctor had stopped referring patients to me, and, other than this, criticism from my colleagues seemed to be limited to the occasional cold shoulder or sharp remark at a hospital staff meeting.

I felt I had a lot to be thankful for. As a physician my days were ever more gratifying, and for the first time I could say the same thing as a private man. Paula's beauty and quick wit had brought a warmth and vitality into my life that I'd never known before. Her interest in medicine and passionate commitment to the underdog gave us a strong common bond that never ceased to surprise and please me. Hard work was something we both enjoyed, though at this period there was still time for relaxation as well.

On one memorable and, thank heavens, unique occasion, I recall my work merging with my off-duty pleasures in a curious way. I was particularly keen on cross-country horseback riding and know few thrills comparable to that of being on a good hunter, jumping fences and riding through a blooming countryside. I had a magnificent chestnut thoroughbred, who, unfortunately, developed a large growth on the undersurface of his belly. It was a benign tumor, but it was about six inches long and four inches in diameter and it was unsightly. Why, I thought, should I get a veterinarian to operate when I was perfectly capable of removing the growth myself? So I prevailed upon the hospital's operating supervisor, a very capable, good-natured girl, to help me. Dorothy made up an instrument tray, and one hot day in the middle of July we went out to the stables. In the midst of innumerable flies, while the stableboy, who was the third member of our operating team, held one of the horse's hind legs so he couldn't kick, Dorothy and I took out the tumor. We were both covered in blood, sweat and tears by the time I had closed the incision with the heaviest sutures I could find. The next day the man who ran the stables called me to say the stitches had all broken. Dorothy made up another instrument tray and we went out and resutured the incision with steel wire, thinking this could never break. To my chagrin I received another call telling me the sutures had broken again. With belated humility I arranged for a veterinarian to take over, and with further humility I have to admit that *his* sutures did not break.

In my midsixties, I felt about my new life that same kind of joyous exhilaration I had known out in open water, sailing on a good fast reach off the Maine coast. It was inevitable, of course, as my friend Daniel had predicted, that I should run into some squally weather. It all began when I went to Kentucky to testify in the case of a forty-three-year-old man whose gall bladder operation led to bungling of such magnitude that it cost him his life.

Samuel Mitchell was a farmer who lived with his large family on a farm outside the small town of Larkville. After he had suffered several severe attacks of pain in the upper right abdomen, his family doctor suggested a gall bladder X ray, which, not surprisingly, revealed stones. Mr. Mitchell, after further consultation, decided to have surgery and put himself under the care of Dr. Jenkins, one of Larkville's two surgeons. He was admitted to the local hospital, standard preoperative studies were done, and Dr. Jenkins removed his gall bladder.

On the first postoperative day Mr. Mitchell began, according to Dr. Jenkins' deposition, "to experience problems." He had a fever, rapid pulse, respiratory difficulty and was "slightly disoriented." Over the next hours "the patient appeared to be getting worse." He was "sweaty." He was "a little more out of his head." Yet not even when Mr. Mitchell, draining bile from his incision, began to go into shock was the surgeon capable of diagnosing this obvious and rapidly fatal type of bile peritonitis. Nor was this the extent of Dr. Jenkins' ineptitude. An uncertified surgeon because he'd become, in his words, "involved in practicing and did not ever take the examinations," Dr. Jenkins also showed extreme carelessness in giving Mr. Mitchell the near-maximum dosage of a drug called Garamycin. This potent antibiotic is ototoxic and nephrotoxic and can, unless carefully monitored, cause deafness and ruin the kidneys. When the Garamycin treatment began, the day after the operation, the patient's kidney function, as determined by a test called blood urea nitrogen, BUN, was a normal 16. After forty-eight hours of the antibiotic Mr. Mitchell's BUN had doubled. But not then, nor in the next several days as the BUN steadily, alarmingly increased, did Dr. Jenkins stop the drug or reduce its dosage. On the fifth day, when the patient's BUN was around 150, he developed kidney failure and was transferred to a larger hospital where there were facilities for hemodialysis, a method by which the blood is cleansed of waste products. Shortly after his admission, despite intensive treatment, Samuel Mitchell died, leaving a wife and seven children.

All this was sorely troubling me in the days before the trial. It's a habit of mine, when distressed, to begin an obsessive hunt for books about the Civil War, my favorite period of American history. I was in a downtown bookshop one Saturday afternoon when I bumped into Michael Waring.

"Well, you're looking like the professor who can't remember where he left his head," he greeted me. "How've you and Paula been?"

"Terrific, working hard as usual. We'll all have to get together soon."

"How about having a drink now?" Relaxed and tanned even in midwinter, Michael looked more like a tennis bum than the serious hard-working attorney he is. "Or don't you have the time?"

"Sure I do. Let's go somewhere quiet, though."

Michael talked about his mother-in-law, the weather and, of

course, his tennis game until we were sitting opposite each other in a dim quiet corner of the Warwick Bar. Then, lighting one of his thin cigars, he looked at me shrewdly. "How are things going?"

"I'm flying down to Kentucky to testify. A simple straightforward gall bladder operation, and, due to the most astonishing stupidity and negligence, a relatively young man with a wife and seven kids is dead." I took a sip of my drink. "So I'm going on the stand as an expert witness for the plaintiff."

Michael watched me through his cigar smoke. "How many times have you testified now, Dick?"

"Four or five, why? You, of all people, can hardly qualify for the role of disapproving friend."

"I wouldn't dream of trying," he said, with a grin. "I can count on one hand the surgeons of your caliber who are willing to testify for the plaintiff. One finger is more accurate. But that doesn't mean I don't worry about you."

"Oh, come on, Mike. I've handled myself fairly well in court."

"You mean you've been handled fairly well. The defense lawyers have been very polite. Respectful of the illustrious surgeon with his impressive qualifications, right?"

"I suppose so, yes."

"Well, my friend, the velvet gloves are about to come off. Count on it. A few times you're allowed to play the errant knight— nobody's going to get *too* upset. But from now on you've got to watch your step, Dick. Those defense lawyers are going to go after you like you're Public Enemy Number One."

I shrugged, a casual gesture that belied my feelings. I didn't, after all, want trouble any more than any other man. "Listen, Michael, I'm not that naïve. I knew what I was getting into from the beginning. And I did it damn reluctantly, as you may well remember. But now, well, nobody could dissuade me from testifying for the Mitchell family. I think any surgeon I know would condemn the actions of this doctor."

"Sure they would—but in a courtroom? That's always the point one comes back to, isn't it?"

I sighed. "I guess the only point is I'm mad as hell about this case and I'm damn well going out there."

Michael laughed. "I only wanted to warn you, Dick. But maybe I should be warning them."

A week later I was sitting in the courtroom in Larkville, Kentucky. A rather dim room, it was oddly lit by thin shafts of sunlight coming in through small high windows, and, as I watched the judge and the jurors, all of whom had the same dour, guarded expression, I remember thinking that dark and narrow must be the dominant characteristic of the town. The only people in court who didn't, in fact, have this look of unfriendly suspicion were the plaintiff's lawyer, young Mr. Farnsdale, and the plaintiff herself, whom I saw for the first time that morning. A heavyset woman wearing a loose black print dress, Mrs. Mitchell sat wedged in the pewlike bench with five of her seven children, listening uneasily to the proceedings.

Though I'd read the depositions of Dr. Jenkins and his witnesses, I was nonetheless shocked by the testimony I heard. The defense lawyer, a short, stout fellow named Will Sherman, steering clear of the important medical issues, tried to blame everything that happened to Samuel Mitchell on a "stroke." Two local physicians agreed, under oath, that Dr. Jenkins' professional conduct had been exemplary. As for the defendant, a seemingly relaxed middle-aged man in a neat seersucker suit, he made a lot of general statements to the effect that (a) he wasn't sure that bile peritonitis could cause any real problems, (b) the patient's rapid pulse, mental confusion and spiking temperature were the result of a stroke, (c) the stroke caused the shock that caused the renal breakdown, and (d) if everything in medicine went according to the book it would be real easy.

When I was called to the stand by Mr. Farnsdale he questioned me in great detail, and, as it was crucial that the jury understand exactly what went wrong, my replies were as painstakingly clear as his questions. Despite a growing awareness of the amused glances the defense attorney was ostentatiously exchanging with his client, I tried to keep calm and composed. I explained that the patient's fever and rapid pulse could not have been the result of a stroke but were, in fact, the symptoms of a biliary peritonitis that required immediate surgical care and that, untreated, very probably was the cause of the stroke. I further stated that Dr. Jenkins' negligence had been compounded by his continuing misuse of the nephrotoxic Garamycin, which, in my opinion, had been the direct cause of Mr. Mitchell's kidney failure and subsequent death.

There was a short recess at noon, and before Mr. Farnsdale and I went across the street to the drugstore for a sandwich and a milk shake, we had a brief conversation with the Mitchell family near their truck in the courthouse parking lot. The younger children hung back, but Mrs. Mitchell and her two teenaged daughters asked shy, solicitous questions about my accommodations at the motel and thanked me for coming to Larkville.

"I only hope it does some good," I said, unable to conceal my distress at the morning's proceedings.

"Come on, you all, cheer up, now," young Farnsdale said with a kind but palpably false heartiness. "We've still got a fighting chance."

Well, as it turned out, when the court reconvened and I was called back to the stand to be questioned by Mr. Sherman, there was a lot of fighting and very little chance. Not only Michael but Paula too had said that sooner or later the defense lawyers were bound to get rough with me; that it was a common tactic to distract the jury by trying to destroy the credibility of the plaintiff's witness. But no matter how prepared I thought myself, in truth, I was completely stunned by Mr. Sherman's attack. Under his cross-examination the focus left the defendant doctor whose malpractice had led to a patient's death, and suddenly it was I, the expert witness for Mrs. Mitchell, who was on trial.

Mr. Sherman's line of questioning skittered along the surface of the case, and when occasionally I was able to bring out a medical fact he'd glance over at the jury with a knowing smile. The one point that most interested him and which he kept rephrasing in his soft sarcastic voice was why had a surgeon from Philadelphia seen fit to come all the way down to Kentucky? Though in time I grew accustomed to vitriolic attacks from defense attorneys, I've never forgotten my dismay, the heat of my embarrassment, at this first volley of accusatory questions, which I truthfully, and with what dignity I could muster, denied as fast as they were thrown at me. Don't I advertise my services as a plaintiff's witness in legal journals? Isn't it true I'm always available to come to court for anybody who wants me? Don't I, in fact, make my living testifying for the plaintiff? And the climactic "How much do you charge for your testimony, Doctor?"

During this cross-examination I saw the dispassionate faces of the jurors become openly hostile, and though the plucky Mr. Farnsdale tried, under a redirect examination, to bring the focus back to medicine, we both knew that we had lost the fight.

To clinch the case, Mr. Sherman in his final summation carefully avoided any mention of Garamycin or Mr. Mitchell's kidney failure. Instead he emphasized the testimonial praise of the defendant's two local witnesses and admonished the jurors to remember that not only had Dr. Jenkins been practicing medicine in Larkville for twenty-five years but his daddy, Dr. Jenkins, Sr., had taken care of everybody in town for years before that. Surely they weren't going to bring in a verdict against the defendant on the testimony of a stranger from Philadelphia?

It took the jurors less than an hour to come back with a verdict completely absolving Dr. Jenkins in the death of Samuel Mitchell.

The Mitchell case marked the end to the calm period of my medicolegal activities. My reception at medical meetings grew distinctly cooler. In the operating-room lounge more than one colleague confronted me with a straightforward "You're a traitor to your profession." A gynecologist friend not only stopped referring patients to me but made a point of dropping out of the monthly bridge game a group of us had been getting together for since we were interns. And Daniel Haber told me that my "courtroom activities" were provoking a censorial chorus at Jefferson Hospital, a kind of "low rumble," as he put it.

Now, at this time, I was still very active at the Albert Einstein Medical Center, at the small suburban Haverford Hospital which I had helped found, and at Jefferson Medical College Hospital, where I'd been a staff member for over thirty years. Though my work in surgical instruction had petered out completely at the latter hospital, I hadn't made the obvious connection—partly because, like most older staff members, I'd been doing less and less teaching, since it was the policy to give the assignments to younger men and to those doctors whose entire professional life centered around Jefferson. Practicing surgeons who teach on a part-time basis at a medical-college hospital are not paid. There's a certain prestige to it and, far more rewarding, a stimulating contact with the students and interns. Though I missed the vital involvement of teaching, I had put my lack of assignments down to a kind of normal surgical attrition, to the workings of the "system."

Dan, uncomfortable in his role of Cassandra, at first refrained from mentioning Jefferson's growing disapproval. Then, one Sunday when Paula and I were at his country place for a cook-out, he managed to coerce me into helping him at the barbecue pit, an insistence I didn't understand until we were safely installed behind his "smokescreen."

"I didn't want to say anything in front of the others. In fact, I've been putting off saying anything at all, Dick, but apparently there was a hell of a reaction to your Kentucky expedition. I guess the official hope was that you'd stop testifying. You must have heard some of the grumbling by now."

"Sure. So that's why you dragged me out here?" I tried waving aside the smoke with the apron Beatrice had supplied. "You mean I've risked asphixiation just to hear this?"

Dan gave me a halfhearted grin. "I get the impression our colleagues are getting mad enough to start hitting back."

"Are you boys cooking supper," Beatrice said, bringing over a stack of paper plates, "or swapping your usual jokes?"

The rest of the evening passed pleasantly enough, with no further reference to the hospital. I had all but succeeded in putting this conversation from my mind when that next Wednesday I received an urgent call from Father Connolly, a Catholic priest who was a longtime patient and friend.

"Dick, I need your help."

"What's wrong, Father?"

"It's my mother. She's having stomach pains, bad ones. I don't think it's the appendix, but I don't know what else it can be."

"Bring her right over to Jefferson, Father. I'll be waiting for you."

An hour later I admitted Mrs. Connolly to the hospital with a diagnosis of an acute small-bowel obstruction. This condition required immediate blood studies, tube decompression of her stomach, X rays, intravenous fluids and urgent operation. As soon as the other modalities were taken care of I called the anesthesiology department. It was by now four-thirty in the afternoon. I said I had an emergency case. I explained the situation and asked how soon I could have an anesthesiologist or a nurse anesthetist.

There was an odd pause, then: "You'll have somebody when it's convenient to assign you somebody," I was told.

I was staggered by this cold, inimical reply. "But, Doctor," I persisted, "I don't think you understand. This is urgent. We're talking about a seventy-year-old woman with a full-blown, probably closed-loop, small-bowel obstruction. She can't wait very long for operation."

There was another pause. "Sorry, Doctor," I was told, "I think you're the one who doesn't understand. You'll have somebody as soon as it's convenient to make the assignment."

That round I got the message, and I slammed down the receiver. There was no time to lose. Mrs. Connolly had to have surgery immediately, and somehow I had to figure a way out of this hellish dilemma. I rushed upstairs to the visitors' lounge where Father Connolly was waiting.

"Father, I'm going to level with you. Your mother has a good chance of being okay if I can operate quickly. But there's a son of a bitch in the anesthesiology department who refuses to get me an anesthetist. I'm persona non grata at the moment and I'll explain why later. What I want to do now, with your permission is— well, Father, it sounds a bit mad, but I think it's our best chance . . ."

"Yes, what is it, then?" Father Connolly asked, calmly.

"Haverford's a little hospital, as you know, but with one call I can have the operating room and the anesthesiologist ready. We'll put your mother in an ambulance and I can have her on the operating table in about an hour."

Father Connolly didn't hesitate. "I've known you a long time, Dick. Whatever you say is okay with me."

The plan worked. Everything was waiting for us, and Mrs. Connolly sailed through the surgery. Sometime around eleven o'clock, after Mrs. Connolly was out of the recovery room and Father Connolly was reassured and smiling again, I took first him and then myself home.

"You look ready to drop, darling," Paula said. "Did you get any supper?"

"Father Connolly and I had the cafeteria special—Heaven help us, as the good father said."

"That smile isn't fooling me for a minute, you know. What happened? Difficult surgery?"

"Difficult, yes, but not in the usual sense," I said, and summed up the day's events for her. Now that Mrs. Connolly was safe and I had time to react to my brush with the anesthesiology department, I found myself too weary to be anything but depressed. "I still can't believe they'd do a damn-fool thing like that—risk a patient's welfare because they are mad at another doctor."

"Well, it certainly qualifies for the category of outrageous professional behavior," Paula said, coming out of the kitchen with a glass of warm milk. "Here's a well-deserved nightcap. Go on, Doctor, drink it, it's very soothing."

"I suppose I'm really getting into the fray now."

Paula gave me a wry smile. "I'd say that was a fair assessment of how things are," she said, and sat down on the floor by the fireplace, arms wrapped around her knees. "That, by the way, was the second nasty little story I heard today. Michael told me about a neurosurgeon in a New Jersey hospital who had agreed to be a plaintiff's witness. The head of the department got wind of it, called him in and told him if he testified he would be out on his tail and replaced within five minutes. But the neurosurgeon had been expecting just such a confrontation and had gone armed with a tape recorder in his pocket." Paula sighed, staring into the last flickerings of the fire. "A queer kind of battle, isn't it? Doctors fighting doctors. To think, when I was a medical student I really believed it was all about doctors fighting disease." She grinned, came over to give me a kiss and, with that humor that always lifts my spirits high, said, "As for you, Dr. Chodoff, you'll probably go down in the annals of medicine as the only surgeon who had a patient transferred for operation from a large medical-school hospital to a small suburban one."

5

CALLS WERE NOW coming to me from lawyers all over the country, and in addition to my surgical practice I had to allow for the serious time that reviewing medical files demanded. There is a great deal to be carefully studied, beginning with the patient's history and the record of his original examination. If, for example, he had abdominal pain for two weeks and was in the doctor's office half a dozen times without a white-blood count done, or a surgical consultation, and if this is a patient who died of a ruptured appendix after a few days, it is of prime importance to read the doctor's original office records. More times than I care to remember I have seen additional notes obviously scribbled in the margin after suit has been started, self-serving notes that try to excuse the physician's mishandling of the patient. There are X rays to examine, laboratory studies to go through, and the doctor's progress notes and the nurses' notes to study and compare, for far too often they reveal inexplicable discrepancies.

I then write a complete report, usually including abstracts from surgical literature for the attorney. If it's a case in which I find absolute evidence of malpractice, and agree to go to court, the attorney will ask me to give a deposition. It frequently takes a year or so for the deposition to be set up, either in my office or in an attorney's office where there is a court reporter, the defense attorney, the plaintiff's attorney and myself. Following the deposition a further lapse of time occurs which can vary from months to several years. Then many of these cases, not infrequently on the basis of my report or testimony at deposition, are settled out of court. Sometimes the defense attorney agrees that there has been malpractice but the doctor will not permit him to settle. Other times the defense attorneys will simply refuse to make any reasonable offer of settlement and the plaintiff's attorney is forced to bring the case to court trial.

The average patient tends to think that good surgery refers solely to the ability of the surgeon to cut and sew. His technical skill is, of course, essential, but to bring any major surgical procedure to a successful conclusion there must also be a high level of competency in the preoperative routines, the work of the anesthesiologist and the postoperative care.

Good postoperative care begins with the anesthesiologist's watch over the patient immediately after the operation, while he's still on the operating table. It includes his safe delivery into the recovery room and his careful monitoring by the recovery-room staff. If the patient is quite ill, he will then receive special attention in the intensive-care unit; otherwise, he is returned to his room to be observed by the nurses on the floor and the resident doctor.

The vast majority of patients receive adequate postoperative care. Sometimes it is excellent and its quality exceeds the surgical procedure. But, unhappily, exceptions do occur, and these cases of neglectful, often shocking postoperative treatment began to come to my attention.

One such case concerned Rosa Annunzio, a forty-five-year-old woman who entered the hospital for a hysterectomy and, due to constant neglect and mishandling, ended up in a psychiatric ward. It was Jeff Gable, a lawyer in Miami, Florida, who telephoned to ask me if I'd review Mrs. Annunzio's file. He was a complete stranger to me then, but after our talk that day I knew that we would become good friends.

"It just bowls me over what those characters, in the guise of administering angels, did to that poor woman," he said. "Now, I don't pretend to be a scientific man, Doc, but even I can tell that was pretty bad medicine—just from the stink of it."

"Mr. Gable," I interrupted, uneasy at his approach, "I'd have to study the records very carefully before I have any idea of whether malpractice is involved."

"Why, sure you do, but there's no way you're going to believe what went on in that institution, not even when you read it. If you'll read it. Now, I reckon I've got to put things on the line here. I need an expert and a real reputable surgeon like yourself to help Mrs. Annunzio. Though even then I don't know whether my chances in court are going to be any better than a snowball's in hell. Folks around here, my colleagues, figure I'm butting my head against a brick wall. I say, Take it easy, boys, the brick wall's not getting hurt none, is it?" There was a pause. "Well, the fact is, Doc, we're probably up against more than malpractice. Rosa Annunzio's a Cuban woman, so we got us a little prejudice thrown in for free."

"I see."

Jeff Gable gave a deep chuckle. "I doubt it, Doc. Not from where you're sitting up there. I tell you, she could have been a sack of dirty towels for all the attention they gave her. Well, I hate to see them get away with it, you know what I mean? I figure she's got as much right to get well as anybody else. Now about sending you that file?"

"Yes, please do," I said. "As soon as I've studied it I'll let you know what I think."

Rosa Annunzio's medical charts arrived the following week, and, as Jeff Gable had foreseen, it was very hard for me to believe the facts of the case even when they were laid out on my desk.

Mrs. Annunzio was admitted to a city hospital for a vaginal hysterectomy on July 13 of the preceding year. On the morning of July 15 she was taken to the operating room, and surgery was performed by Dr. Hinckley. Postoperatively the patient ran a fever and complained constantly of abdominal pain, but apparently no physician bothered to examine her abdomen. On the fourth postoperative day, though she had pain and a temperature of 101, she was sent to the physiotherapy department for whirlpool baths. The nurse's note read: "Patient had a slightly elevated temp. and complained of chills upon presentation to the dept. Patient has since refused Rx stating 'It made me worse instead of better.' "

The following day Mrs. Annunzio's fever went up to 103. She

was given narcotics and sedatives, but despite her continual complaints of abdominal pain she remained unexamined. There is no record of the attending physician's progress notes until July 22, a week after the operation. At this time Dr. Hinckley wrote: "Patient dry and not moving much, spasms all over for the last 10 hours. Wants Librium."

On July 23 Dr. Hinckley called in a doctor from the psychiatric department for a consultation of what he termed the "psychotic" behavior on the part of Mrs. Annunzio. This doctor's diagnosis was "post-op hysterectomy with fever and psychosis. Psychoneurosis." He prescribed more Librium and Thorazine and recommended the patient be transferred to another hospital.

Dr. Hinckley discharged Mrs. Annunzio with this note: "Rather stormy post-op course. On the eighth post-operative day patient became psychotic and hysterical and was transferred to St. C's Psychiatry Ward."

Upon admission to the psychiatric service of a Dr. Bern the patient was recorded as having "hallucinations." There was also a note that her white-blood count was 24,700. Though this was unusually high and strongly indicative of trouble, it stirred no more interest in her attending psychiatrists than it had in her physicians. Over the next two days Dr. Bern simply observed that Mrs. Annunzio had apparently been oversedated and was now becoming more responsive. Another psychiatrist wrote that "the patient did not seem psychotic."

By July 26 Mrs. Annunzio's rectal temperature was nearly 104, and the nurse on duty noted that the "patient moaned and groaned with each respiration and was perspiring profusely." At this point Dr. Hinckley finally decided that his patient might have a pelvic abscess and inserted a vaginal catheter as a drain, which subsequently produced copious brown drainage. A doctor from the Infectious Disease Service who examined the patient on the next day agreed that she had a pelvic abscess and gave suggestions as to antibiotic therapy. He also noted that she had "diffuse abdominal tenderness" and was to be watched for "generalized peritonitis."

But not until July 28, after almost two weeks of pain and fever, was the patient at last reoperated upon and found to have a peritoneal cavity full of pus. Though Mrs. Annunzio had still to endure a stormy and painful course of recovery, she did survive her atrocious handling.

It appeared quite evident to me that the peritonitis was caused by a bowel injury that occurred during the course of the hysterectomy. In any hospital that kept to even the most minimal accepted standards of care, Mrs. Annunzio would have been examined immediately upon her complaints of pain, and the typical symptoms of generalized peritonitis following a vaginal hysterectomy would have been promptly recognized and treated. Instead she was heavily sedated with Thorazine and Librium, was called a psychotic and was transferred to a psychiatric ward where a further five days passed before her true diagnosis was appreciated.

I called Jeff Gable and told him that I thought this case did indeed reek of "bad medicine" and that he could count on me to stand up in court and say so. I then wrote my report, stating in no uncertain terms my opinion of the gross stupidity and cruel indifference with which Rosa Annunzio had been treated. It was very gratifying to me to learn subsequently that the case was being settled and the patient was spared the further discomfort and humiliation of having to go to court.

One of the strangest cases of postoperative negligence I reviewed involved a sixteen-year-old girl and was referred to me by Paula.

"Will you please study the file and tell me your opinion, Dick? It's a mystery story," she added grimly. "A young girl is admitted into a perfectly good San Francisco hospital and operated on, her parents are waiting, nurses and doctors are around, but for a crucial period of time there's no record of where the *patient* is."

Reading young Marcia Richardson's hospital records was indeed like trying to unravel a most curious, and ultimately tragic, set of events. She was admitted to the hospital under the care of Dr. Franklin with a diagnosis of a diseased left kidney. The day after her admission Dr. Franklin performed surgery. His operative note recorded that the left kidney was removed none too easily but that both the postoperative condition and the prognosis were good.

The nephrectomy as described by Dr. Franklin was obviously difficult. As it was not possible to isolate the renal vessels for the preferred method of individual ligation, mass ligation and suture had to be done. Postoperative bleeding from any organ, including the kidney, is far more likely to occur after mass ligation. For this reason, specific orders should have been written to monitor the patient's vital signs frequently, to record her urinary output, do serial determinations of the hemoglobin and hematocrit, and keep blood available for transfusion.

At 2:05 P.M. Marcia was taken from the operating room to the recovery room. At 2:30 P.M., the recovery-room note stated, a catheter was inserted, but there is no record of how much, if any, urine was obtained. At 2:55 P.M. the patient was given Demerol; at 3:00 her blood pressure dropped from 120/80 to 90/50, and at 3:45 she was discharged from the recovery room. The only other notations were that the patient was good on admission and good on discharge and that her dressing had been reinforced.

At 4:50 P.M. Marcia was returned to her room at the request of her mother. But there is nothing in the hospital records to indicate where she was between the time of her discharge from the recovery room at 3:45 P.M. and the time of her return to her room at 4:50. The nurses' first note described Marcia's dressings as intact and the girl as moaning and complaining of pain, shortness of breath and her eyes "burning." At 4:55 an attempt was made to reach Dr. Franklin. He was not at home, and an "emergency" message was left for him. The emergency-room doctor was called twice, but he was with a patient and unable to come up. By 5 P.M. the patient was gasping, her blood pressure was "faint," her color was "mottled and ashen," and her respirations were very shallow. Dr. Franklin was called again. At 5:05 P.M. cardiorespiratory resuscitative attempts were started, and at 6 P.M. the patient was taken to ICU with an endotracheal tube. She was placed on both a respirator and a cardiac monitor, and was described as having clammy skin, no urinary output and cyanotic extremities. At 6:15 P.M. Dr. Franklin arrived and the first of four units of blood was given. Resuscitative measures were continued, and at 6:47 the patient was taken to the operating room. Her wound was opened, a large amount of blood was released, and attempts were made to stop the bleeding by packing. "After many transfusions," the heart stopped at 8:10 P.M.

It is my belief that both Dr. Franklin and the staff of the recovery room were directly responsible for the unnecessary death of Marcia Richardson. The surgical procedure required that she be very carefully monitored. When her blood pressure dropped precipitously she should have been examined by a physician immediately and returned to the operating room for control of hemorrhage. The statement that her condition was good on discharge from the recovery room at 3:45 P.M. is patently inaccurate. She was beginning to bleed to death in the recovery room—a condition that scarcely could be called good.

This case, with its uncontestable and inexplicable negligence, was settled out of court, but the mysterious gaps in Marcia Richardson's records haunt me still. She was discharged from the recovery room at 3:45 P.M. and, according to the nurses' notes, was received in her room at 4:50 P.M. Where was she for the sixty-five minutes unaccounted for? Why were her dressings noted as "re-inforced" unless they had been soaked in blood? How could these dressings be described as "dry and intact" when she was in the process of exsanguinating from massive, uncontrolled hemorrhage? What was the "emergency" that arose between 4:50 P.M. and 4:55 P.M., when Dr. Franklin and the emergency-room physician were called? And why at 5 P.M., when the patient was obviously moribund, had she not yet been seen by a physician?

Another case that was sent to me at this same time, and also, due to colossal postoperative blundering, was settled out of court, and involved a fifty-two-year-old New Hampshire woman named Leila Dawson. Mrs. Dawson was admitted to the hospital under the care of Dr. Alexander for repair of an umbilical hernia and the performance of a jejuno-ileal bypass for severe obesity. The patient was five feet two inches tall and weighed 253 pounds, so that the indication for the small-bowel bypass was justified, since the patient had been unable to lose weight by dieting.

Mrs. Dawson was operated upon by Dr. Alexander at 7 A.M. Now, it's no secret to any qualified surgeon or anesthetist that major abdominal surgery in the obese carries with it major respiratory hazards. An endotracheal tube should never be removed in any patient until ventilation is adequate, the patient is breathing well on his own, and provisions have been made for maintaining an open and adequate airway after extubation. This patient, massively obese and under general anesthesia for over four hours, was extubated, placed on a stretcher, and taken to the X-ray department in order to find out whether or not she had a retained intraperitoneal sponge. Such surgical and anesthetic conduct is appallingly far below recognized standards of good care.

Dr. Alexander's notes, a damning indictment of surgeon, anesthetist and hospital, read like a black comedy.

Abdomen palpated and no sponge located. Abdomen closed. Sponge count incorrect. They had not counted sponges before we started the incision and they did not tell me this. X-rays taken. Machine could not penetrate properly, X-rays could not be interpreted. Anesthetist took tube out (endotracheal). Patient taken to X-ray department. She went into cardiac arrest—vomited and probably aspirated. Mouth to mouth breathing given. We brought patient back to OR and endotrachael tube re-inserted. Patient well oxygenated but no heart beat. Open thoractomy done. Heart flabby. Adrenalin IV 2 cc. Heart restarted but slow. Many medications given and oxygenated continuously. Heart beats eventually became stronger and regular. Chest closed. Procedures continued. Patient to her room. Procedures continued—IV's, breathing machine, etc. Something happened to breathing machine. Repair man called in, respiration done by mouth to mouth method while we were repairing machine. Patient reconnected to machine. Urinary output excellent. 12:00 patient expired. No cause given in chart.

It never occurred to me that talk of my work for the plaintiff was also going along a patient's grapevine until the evening I received an unexpected visit from a young widower. Ralph Dunham was a physical-education instructor who taught in the same Washington, D.C., high school as a patient of mine. It was on the latter's advice that he had impulsively caught a train after school and come up to Philadelphia to see me.

It was after six when he arrived, and I was getting ready to go home.

"Dr. Chodoff," Mrs. Maxwell said, coming into my office and discreetly closing the door behind her, "there's a young man here, a Mr. Dunham."

"I thought we were finished with the appointments for today, Virginia."

"He doesn't have one. Apparently Mrs. Olgive suggested he come to see you and he just got on a train and came." Mrs. Maxwell hesitated, and then said softly, "He seems pretty upset. I said I thought you could see him."

Mr. Dunham was more than upset. He was a very angry young man, and, as it turned out, he had every reason to be. He and his college sweetheart, Abigail, had been married just a little over a year when one day she suddenly developed fever, vomiting, and abdominal pains. Alarmed by these symptoms, Mr. Dunham took his wife to a large Washington hospital, where she was admitted with a tentative diagnosis of an inflamed gall bladder. Though no studies were done, the surgeon, a Dr. Shields, scheduled an operation for the next morning. Less than twenty-four hours after surgery, twenty-five-year-old Abigail Dunham was pronounced dead.

"They never told me what really happened. I couldn't get any kind of explanation that made sense," Mr. Dunham said, his long, thin face showing all the anguish and bitterness he felt. "That bastard Shields, he never took an X ray to make sure about the gall bladder, and even when Abigail was better the next morning he went ahead and operated anyway. I know she was feeling better. I was right there." Young Mr. Dunham turned away, but not before I saw his tears.

"I'm very sorry—"

"Sorry—Jesus." He jumped to his feet and walked over to the window, where he stood with his back to me. "Everybody's sorry, but nobody tells me what happened. It's like they think they don't have to explain anything, like she's just some little patient, so who cares." He turned around, his mouth set in a hard line. "Well, I care, dammit. I guess I will for the rest of my life."

"Mr. Dunham," I began again, groping for the words that could in no way ease his pain.

"Oh, it's okay. I mean I know she's gone and nothing's going to bring her back. But I'll be honest with you, Dr. Chodoff, I don't want them to get away with it, with killing my wife. I feel that it's a vendetta, you know?"

I nodded. "Yes, yes, I do, Mr. Dunham. And I wish I could help," I added gently, "but there's nothing I can do for you. Not now, at any rate. From what you've told me I think there should be an evaluation of the care your wife received—obviously something went very wrong. When the time comes I will, of course, be glad to review the case for you, but right now what you need is a lawyer."

It was the only time I saw Mr. Dunham smile. "Go to a lawyer? On a teacher's salary?"

I explained that most attorneys worked on a contingency basis that made it possible for the average plaintiff to seek legal redress. I then suggested that he speak with Michael Waring, which fortunately we were able to arrange for that same evening.

In due time Michael sent me Abigail Dunham's file to review. Studying it, recalling the grief and impotent rage of her husband, I felt a deep shame for my profession.

Mrs. Dunham had been admitted to the hospital on the morning of November 10 on the services of Dr. Shields with complaints of abdominal pain, fever and vomiting, beginning the previous evening. Her symptoms and the findings of the physical examination justified a tentative diagnosis of acute cholecystitus, an inflammation of the gall bladder that usually occurs when a gallstone has become impacted in the duct of the gall bladder. Though proper medical procedure called for a gall bladder X ray to verify this diagnosis, none was taken and an operation was scheduled for the following day.

By the next morning Mrs. Dunham's pain had decreased, she was no longer vomiting and her temperature was normal. At this point Dr. Shields had good cause to doubt his diagnosis. Certainly now he should have taken the X ray that would in all probability have revealed a normal gall bladder, and canceled the operation. This was not, alas, done, and at noon Mrs. Dunham was taken to the operating room as scheduled. Her essentially normal gall bladder and appendix were removed, and a small extra incision was made to the side for the so-called stab drain.

At 5:45 P.M., the recovery-room notes stated, Mrs. Dunham's blood pressure had dropped from a comparatively normal 140/90 to 100/70, her pulse rate had increased to 130 per minute, she was cold and clammy, and her surgeon, Dr. Shields, had been notified. At approximately seven that evening the patient was transferred to the intensive-care unit. In ICU her blood pressure continued to drop and her pulse stayed rapid. She had pale skin and produced no urine—a finding which is common in patients in extreme degrees of shock from hemorrhage.

A medical consultant was called, but he made no suggestions as to the diagnosis or treatment. "At this point," he wrote, "nothing else to add from our standpoint. Thanks for privileges given to us." At midnight Mrs. Dunham had an unobtainable blood pressure and thready pulse. Though the nurses' notes called her abdomen "distended and hard," Dr. Shields described it as "soft." His final note read: "Situation appears hopeless—continues with cold clammy skin. No blood pressure obtainable despite high doses of aramine and corticosteroids. Sodium bicarbonate has been given as well as normal saline. Pupils somewhat dilated—respond slowly to light." Abigail Dunham was pronounced dead at 5:45 A.M. on November 12. An autopsy revealed blood clots adherent to the gall bladder area and her abdominal cavity filled by a massive hemorrhage.

That Dr. Shields persisted with the operation despite an uncertain diagnosis, and in light of the patient's marked improvement, was reprehensible; his failure to recognize her postoperative hemorrhagic shock in the following sixteen hours, nothing short of astonishing. Progressive fall in blood pressure, rise in pulse, cold clammy skin, cessation of urine output—this is the textbook description. When the patient first showed signs of shock in the recovery room a rapid transfusion of blood would have helped to diagnose as well as treat her condition. Had this young woman then been taken immediately to the operating room for abdominal exploration and control of post-cholecystectomy hemorrhage, as good standards of care demand, she would have been saved.

Dr. Shields' mishandling of the case was compounded by his dishonesty. On the front sheet of the hospital chart Abigail Dunham's death was listed as due to "irreversible shock," a term no longer used by knowledgeable surgeons. There was no mention, of course, that the shock was caused by a postoperative hemorrhage, nor that it could have easily been reversed by proper treatment.

There was no question that the doctor was guilty of malpractice, and the case was settled out of court. Nothing could, as Mr. Dunham said, give him back his young wife, but at least justice did triumph.

6

IT'S AN ODD human failing that no matter what the signs and portents are, we somehow never truly believe in the possibility of the irrevocable loss of a beloved person or place. This was more or less my feeling about Jefferson Hospital. I knew I was in trouble there, but because, like the other men in my family, I had graduated from the medical school and, like my father, interned at the hospital, and because I'd been a surgical staff member for over three decades, I suppose my attachment was too deep to imagine a real severance.

It was Dan, as usual, who gave me a reluctant report of what two other colleagues had heard: to wit, I was headed for big trouble. That low rumble, it seemed, was growing into an administrative roar. Though I could still number a few faithful friends among my colleagues, Dan was, as he'd always been, my staunchest ally. He was totally dedicated to the ethical principles of our profession and agreed with me that a doctor's main concern should be for his patient, not his own reputation. I know he felt it was wrong to deny an injured patient—or his survivors—an honest explanation and some form of redress. Yet even though I had his admiration I still didn't have his total approval. For all his lighthearted manner Dan is basically a scholar, a scientist who has always been somewhat removed from the life he strives to save. I knew that the extent of my personal involvement in the malpractice issue continued to bother him. He felt that the problem ought to be solved in some abstract orderly fashion, and our talks always ended on the same note of argumentative agreement. "Something ought to be done," Dan would say, and I'd reply, "And somebody has to do it."

On this particular day I had stopped by the cafeteria for a late lunch after finishing my rounds. I remember that I was feeling pleased; a patient I was concerned about, a seventy-two-year-old veteran with a mild heart condition, was recovering nicely from the surgery I'd done to repair a duodenal ulcer. That afternoon he had been in the best of spirits telling "blue" war jokes to a middle-aged and blushing nurse's aide. I got a sandwich and then saw Dan at a table with two pretty nurses.

"Sit down, Dick. Well, now that we're four," he said, with a barely perceptible wink at me, "how about some bridge?"

I gave him a mock look of concern. "You know what the night supervisor's going to say."

The girls looked at us as though we'd gone mad, and after they left we burst out laughing. It was an old private joke that went all the way back to our intern days.

"What was that old battle-ax's name, anyway?" Dan said.

"Stella Morris—how could you forget?" I replied, naming the night supervisor who had been the bane of our youthful existence. A rather mean, sharp-tongued old spinster, she had believed that every intern's sole ambition was the seduction of every student nurse, by whatever means possible. One night when Dan and I were on the obstetrical service, there was a patient in labor and we were playing bridge with two nurses as we waited for her to deliver. Well, along came Stella Morris. "You stop that right now," she cried, shaking her finger at the nurses. "Don't you know this is the way girls get pregnant, playing cards with interns?"

Dan and I sat quietly over our coffee for a while, pleasantly fagged at the end of a good day, and then, "Listen, Dick," he began, tugging at the corner of his mustache, "there's something we have to talk about."

I leaned back, as comfortably as one can in a hard straight-back cafeteria chair, suddenly aware of the clattering dishes and the hum of voices around us.

"If I interpret correctly, my friend, that means there's something *you* have to talk about. Okay, I'm listening, shoot."

Dan gave me a small smile. "An appropriate choice of words. Apparently you got some very important backs up the last trip to court. They're calling you a 'hired gun' now."

"That's me—Bugsy Chodoff."

Dan took off his glasses and gave me a close and unusually severe look. "Dammit, man! I'm serious." He lowered his eyes again, and his voice. "I'm talking about the situation here at Jefferson. The rumor is, if you keep it up you're going to get the shaft."

Somehow I wasn't expecting an outright threat, and for a moment it took my breath away. "I see," I said finally, and Dan gave me another penetrating look.

"It's completely unfair, I agree. In fact, it's outrageous. But, Dick, how can you be surprised?"

He was right. How could I be? I shook my head. "I don't know. I suppose the morality involved here really baffles me. I can't get used to the idea that trying to do something right gets twisted around to wrong. Good Lord, whom am I supposed to be against? A profession I honor? We're talking about a very small, a tiny minority, of doctors who are negligent. We're talking about indefensible cases of malpractice, where the doctor is protected by his fellows and nobody gives a damn what happens to the injured patient. Or his survivors."

"I agree with all of that. A lot of us do—nobody wants injustice and something's got to be done about it. But doctors are human, we make mistakes."

"Sure we do, and we carry insurance to take care of our mistakes. So why try to argue that a wrong is a right? Why keep the image of the doctor sacrosanct, perpetuate the myth of the healing god who can do no wrong?"

"Basically I agree. But you always oversimplify things. Of course something's got to be done. We've got to find a method for policing the ranks. And certainly there's got to be some system worked out to compensate the victims of malpractice."

"And meanwhile what are they supposed to do? We always come

back to that, Dan. What happens to these people now? Who gives a damn about some poor guy in some little place you've never heard of out West or way down South? I never did. I never gave it a thought until I reviewed that first case. Then I began to see what the patient's up against. The defendant's colleagues will cheat, lie, anything goes to save a doctor's reputation—including the reputation of the medical profession itself."

Dan sighed at what was, after all, a very familiar tirade. "You want more coffee? Wait a second, I'll get us both some."

I looked around this cafeteria, more familiar to me, I suppose, than my own dining room. It was very hard to imagine severing a lifelong tie with this hospital.

"Here you go," Dan said, back with two more cups of tepid coffee. "Listen, Dick, you know I understand—"

"I'm not sure you really do. How could you? You've got to read some of these files, see the expressions on the plaintiffs' faces in the really bad cases. They look like they're living a nightmare. These upright respectable doctors whom they admire and trust are lying to them, and to everybody else. And the smaller the town, the less chance a plaintiff has, no matter who the expert witness is. A small-town judge and jury *want* to believe the testimony of the local doctors."

Dan gave me an indulgent smile. "I understand why you feel so incensed—believe me, I do. But right now what's the exact point you're getting at?"

"I guess what I'm saying is that there's no way I could or would stop now. No matter how much people at Jefferson disapprove."

"Well, I'm not defending Jefferson's attitude," Dan said gently. "But it's not unique, you know. There was an article in one of the medical bulletins the other day—very threatening stuff. All about stopping physicians from testifying for the plaintiff, suggesting that their hospital privileges be suspended."

I nodded. "I saw it—or one just like it. They're not rare, those articles. And they're always the same. Never any mention of the crippled or dead patient, and not a word, of course, about those eminent liars who'll invent the most esoteric defenses for their colleagues in cases where there is *no* legitimate defense. I promise you, Dan, you'd be astonished at the way some very well-known surgeons are willing to perjure themselves."

"And you think you can beat the system?"

"No, but I think I can fight it."

Dan shook his head. "What can I say? You're a stubborn fool—and a very courageous man."

"Bollocks."

"Modest too," he said, and we both laughed.

I went back to my office after that to do some chart work, but I kept thinking about what Dan had said. If I was called a "hired gun," what was the name for the defense experts, for those prominent, distinguished doctors who came into court and not only twisted the truth but actually committed perjury? Those men who, in an effort to defend their errant colleagues, were guilty of violating not only their Hippocratic oath but the basic ethics of the American Medical Association. I sat at my desk long after I had finished working, my heart weighed down by our conversation.

Five months and one court appearance on behalf of a plaintiff later, I received a summons to the office of Jefferson's professor of surgery. While I had come to accept the possibility of this moment, it still held no reality. I had not visualized the day, had not imagined being confronted with the issue face to face. In point of fact, though, my meeting with the professor of surgery was hardly a confrontation of the issue. He simply announced, without preliminaries or explanations, that he was not going to reappoint me to the surgical staff.

"Why?" There was so much I wanted to say, but this single word burst from me of its own volition.

The professor studiously avoided my eye, busied himself with the papers on his desk and replied, "You're not doing any teaching."

"I can't very well teach when I'm not given any assignments."

There was more shuffling of papers and then my dismissal. "Sorry, Doctor, that's the way it is."

It would be a falsehood to say I was not thoroughly undone by this scene, no matter how well prepared I had thought myself.

Though I didn't really expect he would be able to help me I went immediately to the dean. We had remained friends, despite my legal activities, and to me he was a symbol of the Jefferson I had always known, the traditions that bound me and my family to the hospital. The dean was standing by his window reviewing a hospital chart when I walked in on him. He raised an eyebrow at the expression on my face and quickly put down his papers.

"Sit down." He knew, of course, why I was there. "It's been a long time coming, Dick. I knew they wouldn't reappoint you," he said. "Not as long as you're continuing to testify against other physicians. I'm sorry, but my hands are tied. There's nothing I can do for you." His concern and honest regret helped lessen the blow of his words. "I have no way to restrict the appointment power of the department heads. If the professor of surgery doesn't reappoint you, then I'm afraid that's it. I don't know how you can fight it."

Briefly I did contemplate fighting it. Never in all my years at Jefferson had I been reprimanded or criticized for the quality of my surgery. My situation was paradoxical, to say the least. For in the very act of upholding the principles of medical ethics—

> The medical profession should safeguard the public and itself against physicians deficient in moral character or professional competence. Physicians should observe all laws, uphold the dignity and honour of the profession and accept its self-imposed disciplines. They should expose, without hesitation, illegal or unethical conduct of fellow members of the profession—

I was, according to my brethren, betraying them. I considered the possibility of taking the issue to the courts, for I felt quite sure I could win my reappointment. But it was easy enough to imagine what form Jefferson's reprisals would then take: trouble getting any staff cooperation, no beds available for my patients, and great difficulty in scheduling operations. That evening I discussed the situation with Paula. More realistic than I, she had been expecting this particular boom to be lowered for some time. Though she thought it was unjust, she agreed with my decision not to fight it.

"If you're going to do battle, Dick," she said, "there are, as you and I know, far worthier causes."

The next day I handed in my resignation from Jefferson and in the evening when I got home found flowers and candles on the dining-room table, my favorite, and most expensive, white wine in the ice bucket, and Paula looking especially lovely and festive in a flowered hostess gown.

"When on earth did you do all this?" I asked, flabbergasted.

"I was nearly finished with my research for the new brief, so I left the library a little early."

I stood there frankly puzzled. "But you can't really think this is a day to celebrate?"

"What I think," Paula said lightly, "is what's the sense of celebrating the great things? Who needs it when you're already high?" She opened the wine. "These are the sensible times for cheer."

I had to smile. "Flawless logic, Miss Stone."

Paula filled the glasses. "I thought you'd see it my way." And then, her face suddenly sad and serious, she said, "Oh, hell, Dick. I hate this for you. It's so damned unfair. And I mean for the hospital too, to lose such a surgeon."

"How are you going to like being the wife of a renegade doctor?"

"You know me, I'm going to love it." She paused. "Okay, so now you're going to be really ostracized—but from what? A fraternal society, a closed corporation whose main concern is to protect its own members? What kind of sense does it make that a brotherhood created to help patients should shut their eyes when somebody's hurt by malpractice and worry about helping themselves? At least you've got the integrity to fight for what you believe in, Dick. No matter what they take away, you've got your self-respect. And, God knows, you've got mine." Here Paula flashed me that quick beautiful smile of hers, and the love and pride I read in it not only gave me courage but made me realize that I had, after all, reason to celebrate.

My son Bill and dear Mrs. Maxwell were also quick to rally round with their support. Bill, who had decided against a remunerative private practice in favor of running a home-care program for children in an underprivileged community, was a source of pride to me. It was always reassuring to speak with him about the malpractice situation. A little shaming too. Here I was, only now, in later life, learning to whom my allegiance belonged, whereas young Bill didn't have any hesitation in putting justice, morality and, above all, medical ethics over material considerations.

Once I recovered from the shock of the Jefferson affair I felt a curious relief. Naturally, it continued to distress me, as it still does, that a doctor's concern for the maltreatment of a patient can be construed as treachery to the medical profession. Yet I was stubborn enough to be glad the fight was out in the open. A few more angry colleagues began shunning me, and still another stopped referring patients. By now, of course, there was an appreciable decline in my income, though not enough to change my way of life. Or perhaps, as Paula pointed out, my interests and priorities had already changed. Oh, I still liked sailing and trips abroad whenever possible, but there seemed to be a curious reversal to my life: the older I was getting, the harder I worked. In addition to my private practice, I began concentrating my energies on my staff work at Haverford Hospital, and, of course, I continued strong with my medicolegal activities.

The defense lawyers' personal attacks ceased to bother me. I learned how to become hydra-headed; each time my head was chopped off I grew a new one. I discovered that the court is an adversary ground, full of attacks, counterattacks, brilliant and sometimes stupid legal maneuvers. Experience taught me that the more indefensible the defendant doctor's actions, the fewer medical facts are mentioned and the more concentrated the attacks on me: first, to make the jury think that my testimony is for sale; secondly, to get me angry. A witness who has lost his temper becomes easily flustered and can be forced into untenable situations. I made certain rules for myself: always to tell the truth; to try not to lose my temper; and whenever I didn't know something, to admit it.

It continued to surprise me how easily the defendant doctor could surround himself with colleagues who were determined to protect him at all costs. In 1976 I testified in three trials and at each one found myself startled and appalled at the testimony given by the defendant doctor's expert witnesses.

The first case involved a woman of thirty-eight named Gail Rogers. She was an executive secretary, a single woman with some emotional problems that tended to manifest themselves in physical complaints. Living in a large Southern city where there were several hospitals and a well-known medical school, she made the usual medical rounds common to some psychoneurotic patients. Many studies were made, but no organic basis for her complaints was found. Finally, in one hospital, as some of Miss Rogers' symptoms were gastric a gastroscopy was decided upon, and a tube was passed down the esophagus to enable the doctor to visualize the interior of the stomach. After this procedure the patient was returned to her room.

Within several hours she had a temperature of 101 and was complaining of chest pain and difficulty in swallowing. A review of Miss Rogers' chart showed the classic signs and symptoms described in all surgical texts as typical of perforation of the esophagus in the chest by the instrument, a recognized hazard of gastroscopy. Repair of the man-made hole can be accomplished surgically if the patient is operated on within twelve to eighteen hours, but diagnostic and therapeutic measures must be started instantly. One of the most important orders in such a case is that the patient be given nothing by mouth. Any material contaminated by the bacteria in the mouth could, once swallowed, pass through the hole in the esophagus and produce a virulent, and sometimes fatal, infection within the chest. Incomprehensibly, the obvious diagnosis of perforation was neither made nor even suspected. The patient's symptoms were assumed to be gastritis, and she was given large quantities of liquid antacids and milk at frequent intervals.

For one full week Miss Rogers, suffering from high fever and extreme chest pain, was maintained on this routine. The material collecting in her chest produced a massive, foul infection. Her chest cavity was full, not only of pus, but of the milk and antacids that had been given to her every hour. At last the diagnosis was made, and the patient was subjected to several trips to the operating room for multiple drainage procedures, and to many months of hospitalization.

Miss Rogers, when finally discharged from the hospital, consulted a well-known trial lawyer, who sent me the records of the case and asked for my opinion as to whether her care had met with the accepted standards. My reply was that while I did not think the original perforation had been evidence of negligence, the subsequent failure to diagnose and treat an obviously life-threatening complication certainly was.

After months of legal negotiations with no settlement, the case came to trial. When I was sworn in as a witness the plaintiff's attorney asked me my opinion of the care Miss Rogers was given, and I replied that I thought it had been abysmal. I explained that the hole in the esophagus had made itself evident very shortly after the gastroscopy, that a surgical closure of the perforation within a few hours would almost surely have prevented Miss Rogers' infections, multiple operations and long hospitalization. I emphasized that the failure to prohibit intake by mouth, and the frequent administration of antacids and milk had compounded the chest infection.

When the defendant doctor's case was presented, two of his colleagues testified that his handling of Miss Rogers had been exemplary. The final witness was a well-known thoracic surgeon, chief of the department in the city's medical school, with a national reputation. His testimony, brief and to the point, disagreed in most respects from other authorities. He told the jury that the way to treat instrumental perforations of the esophagus was to give the patient lots of milk and antacid to "neutralize the acid stomach juices that came out of the hole."

The jury, without medical background, had to base its verdict on obviously contradictory testimony, and it was not surprising that a defense witness so respected in the city helped bring in a verdict in favor of the defendant. Miss Rogers, who had suffered so much from negligence, received no compensation for her mistreatment.

The second trial had to do with the unnecessary death of Sarah Morgan, a forty-five-year-old Detroit housewife. This time the expert witness for the defendant doctor was so zealous in his attempt to save his fellow that he gave testimony disagreeing with his own authoritative word.

Mrs. Morgan had suffered many nonspecific complaints, some referrable to the gastrointestinal tract. When she was admitted to the hospital a series of tests were done, but none revealed the cause of her symptoms. Though all the liver-function studies performed were normal, as one would expect in the absence of obvious liver disease, one significant X ray revealed an incidental finding that was highly suggestive of a cavernous hemangioma, a large blood-vessel tumor of the liver.

Biopsies of the liver are often obtained by what is known as needle biopsy. This is a blind procedure in which a needle is inserted through the abdominal or lower thoracic chest wall into the liver and a small piece of liver tissue is obtained through the instrument. It should never be done when the tip of the needle may pierce a blood-vessel tumor, which can bleed at the slightest trauma. But in spite of the warning by the radiologist Mrs. Morgan's physician proceeded with a needle biopsy of the liver. The patient's pulse became rapid and her blood pressure began to fall. The surgeon, realizing that she was bleeding internally, took her to the operating room and upon opening her abdomen found a huge cavernous hemangioma covering almost the entire surface of the right lobe of the liver. The tumor was bleeding profusely from the point where the needle had entered it. In spite of all efforts, Mrs. Morgan died in midafternoon with her abdomen still open, her hemorrhage still uncontrolled.

The following is excerpted from my testimony as the expert witness for the plaintiff.

Q. Have you ever performed surgery upon the liver during the course of your career?
A. Many, many times.
Q. Have you performed any surgical biopsies?
A. Many.
Q. Of the liver?
A. Yes, sir.
Q. Is it generally recognized throughout the medical pro-

fession that a cavernous hemangioma is an absolute contraindication to perform this blind needle biopsy?

A. It is a stop sign, a red flag, an absolute warning to stay away.

The expert witness for the defendant doctor was a prominent gastroenterologist from a prestigious clinic in the area. He testified that he had seen the X rays, had reviewed the hospital records and was thoroughly familiar with the case. He was then asked if he saw any reason why the needle biopsy should not have been done. To my astonishment he said, emphatically, no—there was no contraindication. There was no reason, he testified, not to do needle biopsy of the liver in such a situation, and the needle biopsy carried no danger to the patient.

The jury, understandably impressed by the statements of so famous an expert witness, absolved the defendant of any malpractice in the death of Mrs. Morgan. It was unfortunate that the jurors could not have read an article written by this same specialist, which I came across several weeks later, one which dealt with his experiences with needle biopsies of the liver and clearly indicated that hemangioma of the liver, while rare, is a potentially lethal condition if needle biopsy is attempted.

I had joked with Dan about the epithet "hired gun," yet it was no laughing matter. Along with "turncoat," "maverick" and "outlaw doctor," it was a label that we few physicians who testified for the patient had to live with. And what of those who did not tell the truth for the plaintiff but lied for the defense? Such is the misplaced sense of honor in the profession that these men, engaged in protecting a colleague's reputation, are considered above reproach. Any distortion of the truth is not only expected and acceptable but praiseworthy if it helps to get a verdict for the defendant doctor. Even when a malpractice case is lost, no doctor is officially reprimanded for lying, nor, as he was stating his "opinion," can he be tried for perjury.

The most blatant falsehoods I ever heard came from a noted hematologist of a large teaching hospital in southern California. In order to clear the defendant orthopedist on a charge of malpractice resulting in the death of Stephen Waters, this physician blandly testified to the impossible.

Mr. Waters, a forty-seven-year-old car dealer, had been suffering from low back pain for over three years when he was advised to have a lumbosacral fusion. In this surgical procedure the lower vertebrae are exposed, and bone, usually taken from the upper hip area, is placed so that, as the graft heals, the involved area of the spine becomes solidified.

Mr. Waters entered the hospital on May 19, 1973. The necessary studies were done, and the next morning he underwent surgery. On the first postoperative day he was feverish, his blood count dropped and he became jaundiced. As he was experiencing pain far greater than normal for this surgical procedure, his dressing was changed, a large blood clot was discovered, and ice bags were applied.

It was very clear by the twenty-second that the patient's condition was critical and deteriorating fast. His fever continued, his blood pressure dropped, and his blood count continued to fall rapidly. Though he was given antibiotics, they were totally ineffective, and for a good reason. Nobody had diagnosed the complication: an obvious gas bacillus infection, sometimes called "gas gangrene," that produces toxins which destroy red-blood cells and result in acute anemia and jaundice.

According to Mrs. Waters' deposition, her husband called her at work on the morning of the twenty-second and told her, "I've asked for help, but nobody is helping me." He said, "My throat is burning so bad. Will you bring me some antacid?" Mrs. Waters left work at once, picked up the antacid, and rushed to the hospital. She was not allowed to go to her husband's room until the visiting hours began at one o'clock, at which time she found him "all yellow and his eyes were back in his head."

At about this same hour, Mr. Waters was allegedly seen by the hospital's chief of hematology, Dr. Lobel. "Allegedly" because, as gas gangrene produces characteristic changes in the incision, had Dr. Lobel actually removed the patient's dressings and observed the operative area, as he claimed, he surely would have recognized the infection and begun the necessary urgent treatment. The incision should have been widely opened and all devitalized tissue excised, massive doses of the appropriate antibiotics given, and, as the organisms responsible for gas gangrene are anaerobic and don't survive exposure to oxygen, the patient should have been introduced into a hyperbaric chamber with two or three atmospheres of oxygen. But no such saving action was taken. Mr. Waters' condition grew steadily worse, and he died late that night.

Though Dr. Lobel left no chart remarks, indicating his examination of Mr. Waters, though there were no notes made by nurses, interns or resident doctors, this eminent hematologist nonetheless insisted that he had examined the patient. When the case came to court Dr. Lobel, under cross-examination by the widow's attorney, testified as follows:

Q. Now, Dr. Lobel, I'm particularly interested in your testimony that you examined the surgical wounds of Stephen Waters. Is that your testimony?

A. Yes, it is.

Q. What time did you examine the wound?

A. It was probably between one—I'm sorry, it was between one or two P.M. or later.

Q. And who was with you when you examined the wound?

A. I do not know.

Q. Did you need a nurse with you?

A. No.

Q. Did you have a dressing cart?

A. All that was necessary was to remove the dressing, and put it back again.

Q. You put the same dressing back on?

A. I believe I did, yes.

Q. What do you mean you believe you did? Don't you know?

A. I did.

Q. And did you replace the dressing with fresh sterile dressing?

A. Yes, probably, yes, but I have no way of remembering that.

Q. Well, now, you just said two seconds ago that you put the same dressing back on. Now you are saying you put a fresh sterile dressing back on. Which is correct?

A. My memory won't allow me to answer that exactly.

Q. Your memory hasn't stopped you from saying there was nothing wrong with that hip.

A. That was an outstanding finding and I recall it.

Q. And you don't know whether a nurse assisted you in removing the dressing?

A. No.

Q. You are saying, Doctor, that not specifically writing out the fact that you inspected the wound, not writing it out as part of the hospital record, nor any nurses' notes, to the effect that that dressing was disturbed, and put back on—that this is a normal approach to the examination and treatment of a patient. Is that correct?

A. There is a one-page written note here, with all of the pertinent findings.

Q. Right.

A. And I feel I have omitted nothing which is in any way helpful to the patient's course.

Q. Haven't you omitted one thing, Doctor, about that hip? Haven't you omitted one more thing about that hip, when you examined it?

A. What finding is that?

Q. Where have you noted hematoma, Doctor? Didn't you see a hematoma when you took the bandage off that hip?

A. No, I did not think that the wound was inconsistent with a two-day-old operative site.

Q. Do all wounds have large hematomas which require ice bags, and the orthopedist being called, because the neurosurgeon is concerned about the unusual size of it?

A. That was the day before, sir?

Q. Right, so it's your testimony that it cleared up overnight, by the time you saw it?

A. It's my testimony that there was no abnormal bleeding noted.

Q. Was it your concern about being sued, as a defendant, in this case, and indeed your testimony, now tinged with being blamed for the delay between recommending treatment and diagnosis, which were not found out until late on the day the man died some three or four hours later?

A. That's a very inflammatory statement, and a personal affront.

Q. You may regard it any way you see fit . . . .

In no major hospital is it conceivable that a chief hematologist would examine a critically ill patient alone, unaccompanied by a nurse, an intern or a resident. Nor is it likely that had he done so he could have managed unassisted to turn the patient and remove the dressings from two operative sites, one in the lower back, the other in the hip. Even had he achieved this, it defies all reason to believe that he would then replace the old dressing with the same adhesive and leave without making any notation on the chart.

When I was called to the stand I found myself in the uncomfortable position of having to accuse a physician of an outright lie. But I was so certain that the doctor was deliberately changing the facts that I testified exactly to what I thought, as follows:

Q. Now, do you have an opinion . . . whether the description given by Dr. Lobel that he took the bandage off the wound, and that he inspected it and the manner in which he put the dressing back on . . . conforms to the standard of medical care in this community or any other community?

Objections by Defense attorneys, overruled by the Court.

A. My opinion is that, unfortunately, I believe his statement to be untrue.

Q. Pardon me?

A. I don't think the statement is true.

The jury in this sad case found the defense testimony incredible, the defendant's witnesses were not believed, and a verdict for Mrs. Waters was brought in.

7

MY NOTORIETY AS an anti-establishment man was no longer limited to the medical community of Philadelphia. At surgical meetings in other states, if I was wearing an identification tag on my lapel I was very likely to find myself embroiled in an argument with some colleagues who had recognized my name. The dialogue was almost always the same:

"We hear you've been spending most of your time in court, Doctor."

"A slight exaggeration. I believe I testified exactly three times last year."

"The first time was once too often, if you ask me."

"The issue here," somebody else would interrupt, "is why would a surgeon of your professional standing do it?"

"That's easy, gentlemen. The answer is because a plaintiff who's been injured has as much right to an expert opinion as the defendant does."

If this did not lead to heated words of a more personal nature, the conversation would take a general turn and I would simply be reprimanded for not realizing that the main cause of the malpractice crisis was the legal profession and its greedy, unscrupulous lawyers.

In order to prove the point, somebody was then sure to volunteer the latest story making the medical rounds. Typical was the one about the urologist who was consulted by a couple requesting that the husband be sterilized. The doctor agreed to perform a vasectomy, and when the sperm count was secured from the husband postoperatively it registered zero. A year or so later the husband called the doctor to say that his wife was pregnant. He was furious and demanded an explanation. "An act of God," replied the urologist. The husband could find no coverage for such a catastrophic event in his insurance portfolio. He consulted his attorney and asked whether he should sue his wife for divorce or the urologist for malpractice. The shrewd attorney quickly replied, "Both—but the urologist first. In addition we'll sue the hospital, the laboratory and the pathologist. We can probably get child support from somebody, and we can sue your wife's boy friend under the doctrine of harboring an attractive nuisance. There might be some product liability here also. I doubt if we can sue God successfully, since there's no precedent in Pennsylvania law. Besides, there's no money in it."

It is true, of course, that just as the medical profession has its minority of overzealous surgeons and unnecessary operations, so do a small percentage of dishonest attorneys handle unwarranted claims. Many of these are "nuisance" suits, minor matters that obviously do not involve negligence or malpractice but that a lawyer will pursue simply in the hope of getting a few hundred dollars' settlement from the doctor's insurance company. Too often defense attorneys will advise an innocent but busy physician to settle rather than waste time with depositions and court appearances.

This type of settlement, however, only serves to encourage more nuisance suits. That, at any rate, was my experience. In my first years of practice I permitted my insurance carrier to settle several cases of slight complications not due to negligent care by me, the nurses or the hospital. Though I resented the unjustified claim, I agreed that the charge and the sum involved were too petty to bother with, until a fourth claim was filed against me. Then I realized what was happening and refused to settle. The lawyers who handled these types of suits, learning that there would be no further settlements, dropped them.

Daniel was not exaggerating by much when he said he had been sued because of a patient's postoperative sneeze. One of the suits brought against me was by a woman on whom I'd performed a gastrectomy. She had a postoperative asthma attack that caused a separation of her wound. When this occurred I promptly took her back to the operating room and resutured it. Later I was sued for malpractice.

Another case involved a man on whom I'd operated for a duodenal ulcer. He went home in eight days perfectly well, his back a little bit reddened by the tincture of zephiran we had used when we prepped him. The next time I saw the man, who had not paid my bill, was one weekend when Dan and I were at the Garden State Track and passed him at the hundred-dollar window. After six months, I turned his bill over to a collector, and one week later I was sued for malpractice, for "burns" on his back.

Quite a different matter are those unjustified charges of malpractice brought when there has been a serious or fatal ending to what began as a simple surgical procedure. Devastating complications have been known to come not from negligence on the part of the physician or hospital but from the most unsuspected sources, from medication or equipment considered safe by the then prevailing scientific opinion.

I was involved in one such tragic case. I had performed an abdominal procedure on a woman patient at a time when we were using a certain starch powder before putting on operating gloves, and they were generally saturated with it. My patient's postoperative course was smooth, but within a few weeks her urinary canal was blocked. As a result of an allergy to the starch that was on the gloves, fibrous tissues had apparently formed around her ureters, the tubes that conduct the urine from the kidney to the bladder. The patient, I am sad to say, died of this complication. About a year later the glove company issued a warning that this starch could have an "irritating" effect. A malpractice suit was filed by the patient's family, and the glove company and the powder company settled. Though I was in no way guilty of negligence, I chose to settle also.

One of the strangest cases I was ever involved in took place many years ago and began as a malpractice suit against me and Jefferson

Hospital. The charge against me was dropped, but the plaintiff won his suit against the hospital on the grounds of nurse negligence.

I have always insisted that it is as imperative for nurses to write meticulous progress notes as it is for physicians. It is the only way to preserve the continuity of a case, to insure the patient of proper treatment should another doctor take over. In addition, it is a protection for the hospital to keep these detailed files. What can happen in the absence of nurses' notes is illustrated in the bizarre case of Roy Miller.

Mr. Miller was an extremely obese man of about fifty with a chronic duodenal ulcer that began to bleed profusely. I admitted him to Jefferson Hospital, where we watched him carefully in the intensive-care unit, using what methods were available at that time to stop the hemorrhage. Our efforts were unsuccessful, and in the evening I took him to the operating room. Since his obesity made him a poor risk, the purpose of the procedure was not a cure but solely to stop the hemorrhage and save the man's life.

Mr. Miller made a good recovery but was warned that, as no curative surgery had been done, he might have trouble in the future and should be careful. Within two years he was having severe problems with his ulcer and was not responding to treatment. He was symptomatic most of the time and, being a highly psycho-neurotic person, was a difficult one to treat medically. After a discussion with him, his wife and his mother-in-law, it was decided that I should perform a vagotomy, a procedure in which the nerves that stimulate the formation of gastric acid are cut. In order to avoid Mr. Miller's obese abdomen, which had been operated on before and would have presented technical difficulties, I decided to take the easier, untouched approach and divide the nerves in the chest.

The operation went smoothly and presented no difficulties. However, on my arrival at the hospital the following morning, the nurse came to meet me with the announcement, "Mr. Miller's temperature is up to 106 and he's very lethargic." I ran into the room, took the dressings off his chest and found the incision reddened and swollen, with a sensation of "crackling" when I touched it. This was an indication of gas under the skin and meant that the patient had a gas bacillus infection. As surgical treatment of the wound is urgent in this devastating disease, I called the nurse for a surgical tray, opened the devitalized area to the air, removed the infected muscle tissue and under local anesthesia made multiple incisions in the area to permit the entrance of oxygen. As soon as I had started the patient on massive antibiotic therapy I went out into the hall to tell his wife and mother-in-law what had happened.

"Roy has a complication, a severe gas bacillus infection," I told the women. "We're doing everything that should be done for him. Our professor of medicine is an expert on infectious diseases, and I'm asking him to come in for consultation."

Mrs. Miller said very little, but her mother gave me a meaningful look and in a most caustic tone said, "That sort of infection comes from dirt, doesn't it?"

"Yes, and quite frankly I'm at a loss to explain this." I was indeed distressed and puzzled, as this was the first gas bacillus infection that I had ever seen following a clean, uncontaminated operation in which the intestinal tract had not been opened. The source of the infection, the only one of its kind in many years at Jefferson, was, in fact, never found.

To my immense gratification Mr. Miller made a good recovery and returned home, yet shortly thereafter the Miller family started a malpractice suit against me and Jefferson Hospital. Their major allegation was that a high fever had gone unrecognized for over twelve hours and produced permanent brain damage in the patient. More than seven years passed before the case finally came to trial in Philadelphia. The major witness for the plaintiff was his mother-in-law, whose unprincipled but highly imaginative fancies made for the most fantastic testimony I've ever heard.

She began by stating that I had not informed her and Mrs. Miller of the patient's complication in the quiet corridor outside his room, but that they had been obliged to "fight their way from the elevator through a crowd of doctors gathered around Mr. Miller's door." Further, she declared that I had refused to speak to them and had not told them the details of the patient's condition. But these were only the small peripheral falsehoods. The witness then declared that she had been present in her son-in-law's room when he was brought back from the operating room, that she had seen a nurse go to the windowsill, take a dusty piece of Kleenex and stuff this dirty material beneath the patient's dressing to cover an oozing in the area.

The climax of her testimony, however, was an allegation of malpractice concerning a surgical resident she referred to as "the Oriental doctor." Now, it so happened that at the time of Mr. Miller's operation there was a resident from Japan in the hospital. As this was years ago, he had long since returned home, a fact which made it very easy for the witness to testify that after I had made the multiple incisions in the patient's infected chest-wall area she had seen an "Oriental doctor" enter Mr. Miller's room carrying a large basin covered with cheesecloth.

"I said to him," the witness stated, "Doctor, what have you got there and what are you going to do to my son-in-law?" With a look of mock horror at the jury, she continued, "The Oriental doctor took the cheesecloth off the basin and in it were maggots which he then put into Roy's incisions." Out of curiosity I checked later with the Jefferson pharmacy and found that maggots were last listed available for therapeutic use in the late nineteenth century!

The plaintiff's lawyer next produced a pathologist witness from out of the state, who, interestingly enough, praised my surgery, said I had done nothing wrong, and attributed the infection to the dirty Kleenex alleged by the mother-in-law to have been put over the wound!

I was then called to the stand and examined by the plaintiff's lawyer. As the contention was that Mr. Miller had suffered brain damage because of a high fever undetected by the nursing staff for many hours, the pertinent question addressed to me was, "Didn't you order the patient's temperature to be taken every three hours?" I replied that I certainly had done so and showed the attorney my notes on the order sheet. He asked me then to show him a record of the temperature on the temperature chart. I looked through the file, which was on my lap, found the chart but saw that no temperature had been recorded for some twelve hours. I explained that often when there aren't any graphic records of a temperature there will be very detailed accounts of temperature, pulse, respiration and blood pressure in the nurses' notes.

"Very well, Doctor," said the attorney, "find these notations and read them to the jury." I then examined the record page by page but found no nurses' notes. "I can't find them," I had to admit. Whereupon the lawyer turned to the jury stating that the hospital had deliberately destroyed the nurses' notes to cover up the fact that no temperature had been taken during those hours.

I was then excused from the stand, and within a few hours the judge dismissed the case against me and I was free to go. I learned later that the hospital had a policy of destroying nurses' chart notes after three years; though it must have been known that this case was in litigation, the records had somehow, stupidly, been terminated with the others of that period.

When the case was finally decided by the jury a large verdict was brought in against Jefferson Hospital. As is sometimes done, the attorneys for both sides questioned the jurors afterward as to which witnesses had impressed them and what had influenced their decision—in short, questions that might help them in other cases. It was interesting, though hardly surprising, to learn that none of the jurors believed that a dirty Kleenex had been stuffed under the patient's dressing; nor, of course, did they give credence to the story about the "Oriental doctor." However, they did feel that the hospital had conspired with the record room in destroying the nurses' notes so that nothing could be determined as to whether or not the patient's temperature had been taken during that night.

I do not think that a verdict against the hospital was warranted. It is my opinion that the patient's so-called aftereffects were not attributable to the alleged twelve-hour period of high fever. Although this malpractice suit was unjustified and the testimony of the plaintiff's main witness incredible, the absence of any record showing the degree and duration of the patient's fever left the hospital in a completely untenable position.

The great majority of the files I review represent cases in which complications result in an injury or death despite the correct, assiduous, sometimes heroic medical care by all concerned. A good conscientious attorney, certainly the ones I know, will immediately drop the suit when informed by a legitimate expert that there is no basis for a charge of medical malpractice. I have selected from my files the following letters to attorneys explaining why, in each case, it was my professional opinion that no negligence or malpractice had occurred.

DEAR MR. SMITHSON:

Mrs. Short's case is typical. This patient is one of the extremely difficult cases that occasionally arise when a patient is bleeding from an area of diverticulosis but in whom it has been impossible to determine the exact area from which the hemorrhage is coming.

Based on the X-ray studies, arteriographic studies, and the usual diagnostic work-up, no exact source of bleeding could be found. Accordingly, Dr. Charles did a partial colectomy with restoration of intestinal continuity at St. Mary's Hospital. Unfortunately the patient developed further colonic hemorrhage about four months later. Further colectomy was then done at Central Hospital.

These are extremely difficult cases. The amount of resection done resolves itself into a question of surgical judgment, which, unfortunately, is not always correct. However, I can certainly find no evidence of negligence or malpractice on the part of Dr. Charles.

Another example of progressive disease properly handled by the physician was the case of Hope Munson.

DEAR MR. POWELL:

I have reviewed the records in the case of Mrs. Munson.

Her first admission to Milton Hospital was prompted by: (1) upper gastro-intestinal hemorrhage and (2) gangrene of the toes of the right foot, due to an arterial narrowing that obstructed the blood supply and caused a local anemia. Conceivably the gastric ulcer that was found could have been caused by the frequent intake of aspirin noted in the history. I can find no fault in the care given her at the hospital, although I would question the diagnosis of "a type of Buerger's disease" and would wonder whether or not she should have had an arteriogram or have been transferred to where one could have been done. Whether or not the ultimate prognosis could have or would have been changed is a matter of conjecture. Certainly nothing could have altered the gangrene already present in her toes. The surgical procedures done were indicated and well performed. Whether or not Dr. Sawyer should have requested a consultation with a vascular specialist is not within my province to say, nor can I say whether benefit might have been obtained by such a consultation. My feeling is that progression of her disease was inevitable.

In conclusion I cannot find any evidence of negligence or substandard care in the way Mrs. Munson's case was handled.

The case of Faith Farrell illustrates a common situation in which the patient is anxious to blame the doctor for a postoperative complication that is seldom, if ever, his fault.

DEAR MISS RADNER:

I have gone over the records in the above noted case. This woman had a vaginal hysterectomy done at North Hospital. Her course was complicated by the development of a pelvic abscess which was drained. She recovered and was discharged. A month later she was admitted to St. Luke's Hospital with a diagnosis of adhesive intestinal obstruction, for which she was operated upon, recovered and was duly discharged.

The development of a pelvic abscess following vaginal hysterectomy is a recognized complication of the procedure. In my opinion the problem was handled correctly. It was unfortunate that she developed the intestinal obstruction later, but this certainly cannot be attributed to any negligence on any physician's part.

As for those unprincipled lawyers who might pursue unwarranted claims, I believe there are enough governing bodies and conscientious members in the various bar associations prepared to deal with them. In fact, the legal profession has been far more attentive to its internal policing than has the medical profession. Not long ago, the bar association in a certain state over the period of a year either censured or caused disbarment of sixty-three lawyers. The state board of medical licensure in this same place and during the same time revoked the license of one physician, a narcotics addict who had been the defendant in a number of malpractice cases.

It is an unfortunate fact that though many physicians are aware of medical carelessness or incompetence around them, they will not report their erring colleagues to an appropriate disciplinary board. It is also true that when a hospital discovers repeated negligence on the part of a staff physician it will not only allow him to resign but will also supply him with a good reference for the next hospital.

Dr. Robert C. Derbyshire, a Santa Fe surgeon and former president of the National Federation of State Medical Boards, has given newspaper interviews citing the case of a New Mexico surgeon who performed a gall bladder operation and tied off the wrong duct. The patient died. The error was discovered at the autopsy, but the doctor was neither criticized nor disciplined. A few months later he performed the same operation and made the same mistake, and a second patient died. Again the surgeon was neither reprimanded nor taught how to avoid his "mistake." It was only after the surgeon had lost his third patient under the same circumstances that his license was finally revoked. In short, one has to have a well-established pattern of incompetence before medical authorities will be moved to act. "The philosophy," said Dr. Derbyshire, "apparently is that a man's reputation is more important than the welfare of a patient." The defendant doctor is absolved in sixty percent of the cases that come to trial. When there has been undisputed medical negligence, such as a transfusion of wrong blood, or a sponge or clamp left in the operative site, seventy percent of the cases are settled out of court.

Another complaint the medical profession has against lawyers is the contingency-fee system, the method by which an attorney will undertake a case he deems meritorious without charge to the plaintiff. If the case is lost, as more than half the time it is, the lawyer pays all costs, the plaintiff nothing. If the case is won, the attorney gets a prearranged fee, varying from one quarter to one half of the monetary award. Doctors insist this system is the reason for the increase in the number of malpractice suits, and the astronomical rise in their insurance premiums. The rates depend on the doctor's type of practice, the state in which he works, and whether he has ever been sued, legitimately or not. After each malpractice case, no matter if the physician wins or loses, his rates go up.

That the contingency fee is tempting bait for an unethical lawyer cannot be denied, but the unwarranted suits that find their way to court are relatively few. The costs for bringing a case to court are such that without the contingency-fee system the injured patient of average means would have no chance of finding compensation. To prohibit this system, as many physicians suggest, would be to deny our society's basic beliefs that everyone is accountable for his actions, and that the wronged have the opportunity to seek justice.

And so the arguments chase themselves around in circles: physicians blaming the legal profession, attorneys insisting that the fault lies entirely with inadequate medical care. Meanwhile the patient, about whom the storm rages, is lost and confused. Few win substantial settlements, most receive little or nothing, and the majority don't press suit at all, often because they're too uninformed about the facts of their injuries. As I continued my activities on behalf of the plaintiff I did not see, as I might have wished, the solutions to medical malpractice. I learned only that it is a diffuse and complex problem with varying shades of corruption in nearly every corner.

When I encountered the defendant doctor in court or at depositions, I could usually feel a quite palpable hatred emanating from him. Once in a while, however, I recognized another attitude. I would have the sense of a decent human being who was trapped, who had made a mutilating or fatal error that he would like to admit, settle and try to forget if it weren't for the insurance company pressure forcing him to defend an indefensible case. I would catch a mingled look of confusion and embarrassment on the face of such a man as he listened to a colleague lying for him under oath. When I, as the plaintiff's expert, confront someone like this, my sympathy goes out to him, yet I can't forget the consequences of his error, nor the right of the patient to compensation. As a result, I am so torn apart by my conflicting feelings that I almost prefer the angry doctor who clearly thinks his position sacrosanct and whose uppermost emotion is simply a desire to beat me up. Indeed, once when I was testifying in the South the defendant doctor nearly got his wish. This physician ran what is known as a "Medicare Mill," seeing, very briefly, as many as seventy or eighty elderly patients each day. These hasty, cursory examinations had recently resulted in the misdiagnosis and subsequent death of an aged woman. I gave my testimony to this effect and then went to sit down in the corridor outside the courtroom. When the session was over the defendant doctor walked out and saw me sitting there, and in a rage lunged for me. Had it not been for two of his colleagues restraining him, I've no doubt that that day's legal procedure would have ended in something very like a barroom brawl.

I visited some states where I discovered that an injured patient, or the family of a patient killed by negligence, has enormous difficulty in even finding a lawyer to handle the case. In small towns where the defendant doctor and his witnesses practice, and where the jury lives, loyalty to "their" doctor almost always triumphs over the medical facts of the case. As it is just about impossible for the plaintiff to find a local expert witness; one has to come from a distant city. Distrust of the stranger combined with loyalty to the hometown defendant will usually lead to a verdict in favor of the accused, no matter how flagrant the medical malpractice.

I remember an elderly judge in a Southern town who presided totally helpless at the trial of a doctor whose negligent surgical care had resulted in the death of a young woman. The doctor's father-in-law owned a large mill in town where most of the jury, as it turned out, was employed. Throughout the trial, as each piece of evidence was introduced against the defendant doctor, his father-in-law, sitting there like a grand seigneur, would glare at the jury, daring them to find the accused guilty. The judge did nothing, the jury stayed intimidated, and the verdict, needless to say, was not guilty.

A competent judge will hold his prejudices to a minimum, allowing the trial to proceed with the least amount of fanfare and legal histrionics. But the biased judge is not a rarity, and he can turn a trial into a witch-hunt. He will make the witnesses uncomfortable, the attorneys frustrated and the jury confused by his cacophonic barrage of objections and reprimands. I know of one judge in whose court no competent attorney ever wants to try a case. This man had been a defense attorney, a very poor one, before he became a judge. Once, when defending a surgeon whose bungling had cost a woman both her legs, he argued, "She really has not sustained any real damages because her stumps are of equal length."

Few people realize how much a judge can influence a jury's verdict. His attitude toward the attorneys and the witnesses, his intonations when speaking to them, even his facial expressions, can convey a message. When the judge addresses the jury before they go out to deliberate, his charge to them is often likely to suggest, in blatant or subtle fashion, how he feels the case should be decided.

Judges, like lawyers, like doctors, can be excellent, mediocre or abysmally poor. The quality of a judge is often determined by the character and obligations of the politician who appointed him to the bench. If the court is lucky the judge will be a good one, but this, I discovered, like other luck cannot be taken for granted. One prejudiced judge, for instance, refused to permit me to testify in a case of extreme medical negligence because I did not practice in that particular city and therefore "could not be familiar with the local standards of care." This old "locale" rule, requiring familiarity with local practice, has been revoked in most places, since it harks back to the days when communication was inadequate and medical training differed in some areas. It has no application to modern medicine but is a means of keeping a plaintiff's expert witness off the stand.

The men I came to know best, to have deep respect for, were the plaintiffs' attorneys I worked with: men like Michael Waring and Marvin Ellin whose compassion and sense of justice lead them to take on cases where the odds are not often favorable.

The best sort of plaintiff's attorney is a very careful, studious, undramatic person who will get together with his expert on several occasions before the trial. If Paula is his consultant he will study her medical brief to the fullest extent, familiarize himself with the technical aspects of the particular surgical problem at hand. He is not usually the flamboyant actor; for his verdicts he depends upon a careful analysis of the case, a knowledge of the medical aspects of the testimony, and his ability to recognize when a defendant's expert is obviously covering up for his colleague.

Although I had always considered myself a peace-loving man, I welcomed a new fighting spirit that helped me defend my medical opinions in the courtroom. I discovered it was essential to know as much as possible about the defense attorney—to study his abilities, weaknesses and styles as carefully as a boxer does his opponent. It was sometimes difficult to keep from becoming an advocate rather than remain an unbiased witness giving an expert opinion. The adrenaline begins to flow when the proceedings start, and one realizes why this type of trial is called the adversary system. Dueling with an expert defense attorney is in itself a challenging and often, I found, an invigorating experience.

Since defense attorneys are paid by the hour, unlike plaintiffs' attorneys, they're not often in a hurry to end a trial. In fact, they will often prolong what they know to be an indefensible case with an absurd line of questioning. I was once involved in a case where a young man was admitted to the hospital with typical symptoms of appendicitis. Numerous unnecessary tests and studies were done, all of them negative, yet the simple diagnosis of appendicitis was not made. The patient's symptoms increased: his temperature rose, his white-blood count went up, his pain became worse; and he died. As the insurance company refused to settle the case, it eventually came to court.

The attorney for the defense spent hours quizzing me, going over and over the differential diagnosis of appendicitis. After I had repeated for the hundredth time that in my opinion the diagnosis was simple and should have been made promptly, the defense lawyer, having boxed himself into a corner, said, "Yes, Dr. Chodoff, it's easy enough for you to say this because you have the advantage of the autopsy report."

I think it helped the jury bring in the verdict for the patient's widow when I replied, "Surgeons diagnosing appendicitis, sir, try to make a point of doing it before the autopsy."

I found I had much to learn as I made my way through the

tangled undergrowth of malpractice. One lesson I never forgot taught me the necessity of being more circumspect when speaking off the record with defense lawyers. On this occasion I happened to be involved in two particularly dreadful cases of negligence, both resulting in death, and both represented by the same defense attorney. The depositions were held in my office and were lengthy enough to warrant a coffee break. Since I had met the attorney, Jim Darrel, several other times, and since I considered that anything I now said was off the record, we had a pleasantly informal conversation. I recall very well saying to him, "Tell me, Jim, why are you defending these two murder cases?"

"That's what I'm paid to do, defend, not judge," he replied, agreeing, I felt, that "murder" was the most accurate description. The depositions resumed and were finally completed, and after cordial farewells Jim Darrel left for the airport.

One of the two cases was settled out of court, but the other, involving the death of a young man, came to trial. I took the stand, was sworn in, and on direct examination by the plaintiff's attorney gave my reasons for considering the patient's death an avoidable tragedy. Jim Darrel, the defense attorney, then cross-examined me and, when he was done, rather unexpectedly asked the judge to dismiss the jury. After the jurors left the courtroom, he addressed me again.

"Dr. Chodoff, do you remember the day I took your deposition?"

"Yes, of course," I said.

"And do you remember a conversation we had in the lounge when you asked me why I was defending a murder case?"

This questioning put me in a dilemma which had to be resolved instantly. Since I had not been under oath when making that remark, I could have denied it and that would have ended the matter. But I felt so strongly about the negligence involved in this case that I took the risk.

"Yes, I remember," I replied.

The jury was then recalled, and the questions and answers were repeated in front of them. Since this was a civil and not a criminal trial, it was possible for the word "murder" to be considered an emotional and not factual statement, and, fortunately, this is how it

was interpreted. The jury agreed that an unconscionable carelessness had caused the patient's death and brought in a verdict for the
widow.

As my reputation of maverick surgeon grew, so did the number of
my opponents, for after seven years of testifying they extended
beyond the courthouse and wrathful colleagues to include wary,
vigilant insurance companies. These people, I discovered, were
keeping a dossier on me that contained my depositions and the
transcripts of court testimonies, presumably in the hope that if they
waited long enough I would eventually contradict myself.

Michael Waring, having been the first plaintiff's lawyer I worked
with, tended to keep a protective eye on me. I remember one
occasion when he left an urgent-sounding message with Mrs.
Maxwell.

"What's the trouble?" I asked when I got him back on the phone.

"You, old man. I just thought you should know the insurance
companies are sniffing harder than usual at your trail."

"Well, my insurance hasn't been canceled yet. So they've got
their hound dogs out again—what else is new?"

"The fact that they called Jake Jason to make inquiries about you,
that's new. Wanted to know if he had anything on you."

Jake Jason was essentially a defense lawyer but a good friend of
Michael's and a casual acquaintance of mine. "What did he tell
them?"

"The truth. That you're an honest, conscientious surgeon. But
they won't stop with Jake. So maybe you better think about going
easy, Dick. You know what can happen."

"As a matter of fact, I just read an article written by a doctor who
testified for a plaintiff once. A few days after he was in court he got a
letter from his insurance company saying his policy had been
canceled."

"That's what I mean. And as for you, Dick, these guys are going
to do their damnedest to get anything they can on you. So watch
your step."

"I hope somebody's giving them the same advice."

Michael chuckled. "You're incorrigible, aren't you?"

"So Paula says, but I plead innocent. It's just that when you've been walking around with the sword of Damocles poised over your head long enough you begin to think, What the hell, let it fall."

"That's my boy. Well, frankly, I think Paula and I are right. How's she doing, by the way?"

I laughed. "That's what they keep asking me in court." For Paula had, predictably, become a routine part of the defense attorneys' attacks, and nowadays when I was on the stand I could expect the following sort of sideshow designed to take the jury's mind off the charges against the defendant doctor.

Q. Well, you're a long way from home, aren't you, Doctor?

A. I suppose you could say that.

Q. Your participation as a witness in other cases, have they been on behalf of plaintiffs in suits against doctors?

A. That's correct.

Q. Dr. Chodoff, just how much do you charge for your testimony?

A. My testimony is not for sale.

Q. I assume that you are being compensated for the time you spend in connection with this matter?

A. I am paid, just as you are, for the amount of time I devote to reviewing a case and coming to court.

Q. Are you actively practicing?

A. Actively practicing.

Q. And what is your age, Doctor?

A. Sixty-eight.

Q. Are you familiar with the name Paula Stone?

A. Yes.

Q. She works on malpractice suits, doesn't she?

A. She compiles medical briefs for lawyers, yes.

Q. Will you explain how it is you happen to know Paula Stone.

A. She is my wife.

Q. And in addition to being your wife, what else does she do in connection with medical-legal cases?

A. She is a medical researcher, and I think probably one of the best in the country.

Q. Well, as a matter of fact, doesn't she have a business of working on malpractice cases, and supplying expert witnesses, including you?

A. She doesn't supply me. I supply myself. She gets a lot of files, from a lot of lawyers, and if it involves surgery, for example, she will ask my opinion, Is this, or is this not malpractice, and I will say in ninety percent of the files that I look at, there is no malpractice; and I so advise her.

So she advises the attorney, who so advises his client; and there is no malpractice suit.

Q. Yes, and the other ten percent of the cases, I suppose, exactly the contrary is true.

A. That's correct.

Q. You don't direct her as to how to conduct a search of articles, or anything of that kind. Is that right, sir?

A. My wife had two years of medical college. Her I.Q. is 168; and she does not need directions from me.

Q. How old is she?

ATTORNEY FOR THE PLAINTIFF. Objection. I don't see what relevancy that has to this case at all. I object.

THE COURT. Does it have any relevancy, how old his wife is?

ATTORNEY FOR THE DEFENSE. I think so, Your Honor.

THE COURT. Objection overruled.

ATTORNEY FOR THE DEFENSE. How old is your wife?

THE WITNESS. My wife is thirty-six.

And the defense attorney with a triumphant glance at the jury then dismissed me. Why the difference in our ages is thought to be a secret defense weapon, and why it should destroy my credibility with the jury, Paula and I never quite figured out, but it has given us some merry moments of speculation.

There have been other and merrier moments in our life, to be sure, but inevitably my memories return to the fight, especially to those cases on which we worked together. I remember particularly well the evening when Paula told me about little Peter Franklin, whose case was sent to her by a Minnesota lawyer. We had planned a night out on the town, as we'd both been working rather harder than usual. Paula had been holed up for days on end doing research at the library of the College of Physicians. I'd been away at a medical-education seminar, returning just in time to finish writing an already overdue paper on early surgery for acute cholecystitis. Well, in any event our plan was to take Friday night off, have dinner at an Italian restaurant, and follow the Italian motif through with a Fellini film we'd both been looking forward to seeing. However, when I got home from the hospital I found Paula nowhere near ready.

"I thought we had a date tonight," I said, surprised to find her still at her desk.

"Oh, Lord, Dick, I forgot, completely." And without wasting time on any more of a social exchange, she continued with a resolute, urgent "There's a case. I want you to review it for me."

"Can I take my coat off first?"

"It's no joking matter, Dick. Especially not this one."

"That bad?"

"I think so, but I need to know what you think. I want the best surgical opinion I can get. One thing for sure, it's the kind of file that I get a gut reaction to. When I read something that sends chills up and down my spine, it's usually a case."

"Anything more scientific you care to add, Miss Stone?" I teased.

Paula lunged at me with a mock feint and a smile that quickly faded. "This one's a shocker, Dick. A young couple took their baby to the hospital, a little boy fourteen months old who had, even to my limited medical knowledge, recognizable signs of an internal obstruction. And it was overlooked by not one doctor, mind you, but four. And the result? Permanent brain damage. This perfectly fine little Peter Franklin was turned into a vegetable. His poor parents." Paula's hand went to her breast, an unconscious gesture I have observed often, the reflex that signifies empathetic pain.

Well, we did not, of course, go out on the town that night. I made us some scrambled eggs with mushrooms while Paula gave me a few more details about the case and Peter's young parents,

Bertrand and Rosemary Franklin, whom I was eventually to meet in Minnesota. My opinion, after a careful review of the baby's medical file, was very much in accordance with Paula's. This case did indeed represent a shocking departure from any normal standard of medical care Mr. and Mrs. Franklin had every right to expect.

On the afternoon of March 2, 1975, Peter suddenly became sick to his stomach and began to vomit. By the time Bertrand Franklin, who managed a sporting-goods shop, came home from work, around 6:30 P.M., the baby was drowsy and listless and his eyes were rolling. The young couple, growing alarmed, tried to reach a doctor. It was approximately 7:15 P.M. before Rosemary Franklin got through to a firm of pediatricians, one of whom advised her to take the baby to St. Vincent's Hospital emergency room.

At the emergency room Peter was examined by a medical-school graduate who had just begun his internship the previous month. The intern concluded from his examination that the baby had gastroenteritis, an irritation of the stomach and intestines. He prescribed a Compazine suppository and a light diet of skim milk and baby aspirin every four hours.

On returning home, Peter's symptoms progressed, he continued to vomit and developed a fever, his temperature rising to 102. The couple kept the baby in their room throughout the night. When Mr. Franklin got up and went to work at 7 A.M. on the following day, March 3, Peter was still sleeping. However, at 11 A.M., after being fed some skim milk, he began vomiting again. Mrs. Franklin called the pediatricians' office and received further dietary instructions. When she found that Peter could not keep down either skim milk or cola, Mrs. Franklin called again and this time was told to bring him to the pediatricians' office. He was examined by Drs. Spenser and Niven, who palpated a mass in the baby's abdomen and diagnosed a possible bowel blockage by intussusception, a telescoping of the bowel or intestine. Arrangements were then made for Peter's immediate admission to the hospital.

On the way to the hospital he passed some blood per rectum. The recorded admission physical examination notes that Peter was a well-built white male child of fourteen months who looked quite sick. He appeared toxic and moderately dehydrated, with dry lips, dry skin and sunken eyes. He responded poorly and was pulling his legs up to his abdomen, in bouts, as if he was having pain. His temperature was 104⁴, pulse 130.

At the time of admission, the admitting intern had a telephone consultation with Dr. Spenser and sent Peter to St. Vincent's department of radiology for a barium enema and X rays. According to the radiologist, these did not indicate an intussusception or bowel blockage, although he did see a small rounded shadow which he perceived to be a polyp. He reported these findings by telephone to Dr. Spenser.

On the evening of March 3, Dr. Spenser visited Peter in the hospital and brought in a surgeon, Dr. Martin, to join in his care. Dr. Martin's note of this surgical consultation read: "Barium enema reported large colonic polyp. Patient does not look sick at present. Has round mass in right lower abdomen. Recommend repeat barium enema."

On the following morning, Saturday, March 4, Dr. Martin found that the barium enema had not been repeated, but due to what he perceived to be the child's improved condition, he no longer thought it was necessary.

On Sunday morning, Peter's condition became worse, and at noon Dr. Martin operated. He found a bowel blockage by intussusception with about six inches of intestine gangrenous, which he removed and then rejoined the bowel. The child's postoperative recovery appeared to be normal. His parents went home, but were called back when Peter's temperature soared to 106⁴ due to the gangrene.

Peter went into septic shock and according to Dr. Martin's notes:

He became completely comatose. He had intravenous fluids and steroids for two weeks on and off. He never fully regained consciousness. Felt that he had a considerable amount of mid-brain damage, although he eats and seems to look alright, he does not respond and has no muscle tone and has had for past two weeks episodes of what have been thought to be seizures. Remains in spastic state with clenched fists, tight hamstrings, some arching of back. Has been maintained on thorazine, dilantin and phenobarbital. It is thought there will be some gradual improvement but total amount is not known.

Unfortunately there was no improvement. As a direct result of the doctors' negligence in diagnosing and treating Peter Franklin, the baby suffered permanent and irreversible brain damage. Medical and psychological examinations done when he was one and a half years old describe him as a

totally brain damaged child functioning at the two month level. Prognosis poor for motility. At some point will need institutionalization, it is clear, but it is left to the parents to decide when. Recommendations—A profoundly handicapped child with a poor prognosis eligible and feasible for institutionalization, parents not interested in commitment now.

The trial turned out to be every bit as outrageous as the case itself. I was one of four medical experts for the plaintiffs, prepared to state, unequivocally, that the defendant doctors had failed to diagnose and treat Peter Franklin's bowel blockage in a proper, timely manner. Three of us took the stand; the fourth physician had assisted the plaintiffs' attorney, Alan Bradford, in the preparation of the case but was not called as a witness.

The four defendant doctors had the usual stalwart lineup of loyal colleagues. It was a big cast and one of the maddest performances I ever saw. The unabashed lying of the defendants and their witnesses, the defense lawyer flinging wild accusations at the plaintiffs' witnesses, plus a bizarre interruption of the proceedings made this courtroom not only a gladiators' arena but the Circus Maximus.

According to Dr. Martin, on Saturday, the third day of Peter's illness, he found the child's condition "improved." But Mrs. Franklin testified that she and her husband were at the hospital from 11 A.M. to 7 P.M. and that Peter was, in fact, listless, sick and vomiting. She further testified that during this eight-hour period their son was not seen by a physician. Dr. Martin indicated that he *thought* he saw the child on Saturday night, when he performed an appendectomy at St. Vincent's Hospital, but the hospital's operating-room records showed that no such surgery had been performed on that evening.

One of the plaintiffs' expert witnesses was the chief of the department of radiology in a large, well-known hospital. He testified that the X rays done when Peter first entered the hospital were characteristic of intussusception. Nevertheless the defendants' witnesses testified that the "diagnosis was an extremely difficult one" and that the doctors had handled the case properly.

When I was called to the stand I testified that Dr. Martin's inaccuracies were considerable, beginning with the observation that the baby "did not look sick" on the first day, and that "his condition was improved" on the next. In addition there was his note that the barium enema showed a "large" colonic polyp when the radiologist reported a "small" one. This variance certainly suggested that Dr. Martin had not taken the trouble either to look at the films or to speak with the radiologist. In any case, it should have been perfectly obvious to Dr. Martin that the polyp itself could in no way be responsible for the child's symptoms.

I stated that from the beginning Peter's symptoms had answered the textbook description of a typical intussusception, and there was no possible justification for a group of supposedly well-trained and experienced physicians temporizing and delaying operation until the child's bowel was gangrenous, causing septic shock that led to total, irreversible brain damage.

The defense lawyer then changed the focus of the trial completely by attempting to persuade the jury that the plaintiffs' witnesses had conspired with Mr. Bradford, and his medical adviser Dr. Mitchell, to provide "bought and paid for" testimony. Repeatedly referring to us as "those three cohorts," he tried to inject a false issue into the case by implying that our knowledge of each other, social or by reputation, was a "conspiracy to render collusive and untrue testimony." Questioning the neurologist, the defense attorney asked:

Q. How did Mr. Bradford find you of all the neurologists in the United States? How did Mr. Bradford suddenly call up one day in New York City and say, 'Doctor, come testify for me.

Don't do a darned thing for the baby; don't talk to the doctor, don't find out what's being done for him, just get on that stand and say the baby is going to live forever.' How in the whole world did Mr. Bradford know to call you?

A. I don't know. Ask Mr. Bradford.

Q. Have you talked to any other medical personnel about this case before meeting with Mr. Bradford?

A. No, sir.

Q. I noticed you discussing something with a gentleman in the back; do you know who that is?

A. Dr. Mitchell. I met him last night.

Q. You did not know Dr. Mitchell before?

A. No.

Q. Did you stay in one of the local motels?

A. I did, at the Holiday Inn East, I think it is.

Q. Dr. Mitchell stayed at that motel?

A. I believe so, yes.

The attack on me followed the same pattern:

Q. How did it happen Mr. Bradford contacted you?

THE COURT. If you know.

A. I don't know. I can speculate, but I don't know.

Q. Has he contacted you in the past?

A. No.

Q. This was the first time he had ever contacted you?

A. Yes, sir.

Q. Do you know Dr. Mitchell?

A. Yes, sir.

Q. Have you worked with Dr. Mitchell on numerous malpractice lawsuits?

A. No, I know him socially.

Q. You know him socially?

A. Yes, sir.

With extraordinary persistence and zeal, in the most flamboyant attempt to divert the jurors' attention from the merits of the case, the defense counsel kept up his attack on "these guys, bought-and-paid for witnesses that run around in a group and testify all over the country."

In reference to the testimony of the professor of radiology, the defense attorney ranted to the jury, "Now, why did he come here? He's the head of the Department of Radiology. He's the chief of the department. He says, 'In my hospital we have a specific pediatrics radiologist who does this kind of thing.' Well, if he's the chief, if he's the head, and he really thought something was wrong, why didn't he tell that pediatric radiologist to come on down? Maybe it has something to do with the strange Dr. Mitchell in the courtroom, his social friend who he went to medical school with; the same Dr. Mitchell that Dr. Chodoff knew."

The defense counsel also referred to me as "the fellow that came in here to do my client in. That's kind of blunt, but that's what Dr. Chodoff is here for. . . . Now, I'm not going to knock anybody, but he came all the way here from Philadelphia to do Dr. Martin in."

Then, at the climax of the proceedings, at the end of the trial, when the plaintiffs' attorney was halfway through his summation, the courtroom door suddenly burst open and a man came running into the court shouting, "Is there a doctor in the house? Is there a doctor in the house?"

The four defendant doctors jumped from their seats like a well-rehearsed comedy act and followed the man, who hastily identified himself as an attorney, out of the courtroom and down the hall to where the trouble was. The jury was sent out of the room, and some of the jurors saw the defendant physicians administering medical treatment to a woman lying on the floor of a nearby courtroom.

The judge then told the bailiff to go down the hall to the other courtroom and bring back the defendant doctors. Then he sent the bailiff to get the attorney, whom he promptly placed on the stand and questioned until the situation was explained to his satisfaction. According to the attorney, he had been representing a petitioner in a workmen's compensation case. He had hoped to get her a reasonable sum of money, and when the court awarded his client what she considered an unreasonable sum, she fainted. Frightened

134

by this, and knowing there was a malpractice case down the hall with a lot of doctors, the attorney had come running for help.

When the judge was finally convinced that this was an impulsive act and that the interruption was in no way part of a conspiracy on behalf of the plaintiffs or the defendants, he let the lawyer off the stand and brought the jury back to the courtroom, and the plaintiffs' attorney resumed his closing.

After the summations the jury retired to deliberate upon a verdict. I was subsequently informed that they returned a decision in favor of the defendant doctors. The plaintiffs argued that they were denied a fair trial by the conduct of the defendants' counsel in interjecting improper innuendos of a conspiracy between their counsel and expert witnesses to render untrue and collusive testimony. Their appeal went to the Minnesota Supreme Court and, in a five-to-two decision, they were granted a new trial. The case was eventually settled, and the Franklins were given a substantial enough sum for the future care of their brain-damaged child.

8

THE YEAR ended my sixth decade, a sobering thought. It was in other ways too a year of change for me, a time to reflect on beginnings and ends. The happiest event had to do, of course, with a beginning. Paula decided to enter law school, continuing to work as a medical consultant while she studied law, an extraordinary undertaking that could not have pleased or impressed me more.

Infinitely sad, in this same year, was the death of my first wife, Dean. We had not met over a long period of time, for our divorce had been no more amicable than our marriage. When Dean became ill we saw each other again, and, oddly, there was an easy friendship between us, as when we had first encountered each other, the young doctor and nurse. Only the bedside we met at now was Dean's own and she was dying of cancer. Several times in the latter, painful part of her illness she called me in the middle of the night and I went back to our old home to give her an injection of morphine and stay with her until the drug took effect. We talked only of inconsequential matters. Indeed, she was too weak to speak much, but I sat close to the bed and held her hand until, falling asleep, she would thank me for coming and tell me how kind I was. Her words made me feel even more wretched, and I'd sit there a while longer, watching her while she slept, too heavy with grief and guilt to be able to leave.

Profoundly disturbed by Dean's death, I was grateful for the distraction of too much work at the hospital, for Paula's intensive studying which turned me into a part-time cook. And for my role in the Hammond case, which also took place during this period.

"Mrs. Edna Hammond is on the phone, Doctor." Mrs. Maxwell paused. "She said would I please tell you she's in Philadelphia."

The name was vaguely familiar, but I couldn't quite place it.

"I hope it's all right for me to call you like this, Doctor." The woman's voice held an odd mixture of hesitancy and determination. "Mr. Frommer said he didn't think you'd mind."

Now the name rang a bell. This was Edward Frommer's client, a widow whose malpractice claim I had recently reviewed. "What can I do for you, Mrs. Hammond?"

"Well, I've come from Rhode Island to visit my sister and I wondered if while I'm here I could arrange to see you."

"Why, of course. Mrs. Maxwell will give you a time to come out to the hospital."

There was the slightest pause. "That's where your office is, at the hospital?"

All the timidity I sensed in the woman came out in the way she pronounced "hospital," and I realized, belatedly, the trauma she must still be experiencing over her husband's death. "Tell me where you're staying, Mrs. Hammond."

She gave me her sister's address, which wasn't too far away, and she seemed very relieved when I suggested we meet there the next afternoon.

I wondered as I hung up what exactly had prompted Mrs. Hammond's call. She had been through quite an ordeal, this I knew from her husband's medical files. He had died from an internal hemmorrhage following orthopedic surgery, another victim of substandard medical care. It was on this point, undiagnosed and untreated hemmorrhagic shock, that I had agreed to testify. I also knew that Edward Frommer was having difficulty finding an expert orthopedic witness. Although several surgeons had reviewed the case and agreed with the claim of negligence, not one would go to court. I remembered now Frommer saying what close tabs Mrs. Hammond was keeping on the situation, insisting that he find the best orthopedic surgeon in the country. "She keeps saying they killed her husband and she *isn't* going to let them get away with it. She's absolutely right, of course," he had told me. "But you've no idea what a personality change this is. She was such a mild little woman."

It occurred to me that Mrs. Hammond might be hoping that I knew an orthopedic surgeon willing to testify for her. Would that I did. Perhaps she just needed to be reassured that I was going to be her witness. Or perhaps she just needed to talk to somebody about her husband. The hospital records had shown such negligence that I couldn't honestly imagine what that time must have been like for her and the children. There were two, I recalled, a boy of thirteen and a nearly grown daughter.

Her husband, Murray Hammond, a fifty-six-year-old typographer, had apparently been in good general health except for a painful arthritic right hip which had troubled him for several years. He'd been under the care of Dr. Houston, a prominent Rhode Island orthopedic surgeon, and when it became obvious that conservative treatment was no longer giving relief, his doctor suggested a total right-hip orthoplasty. In this Charnley-Mueller operation, named for its British and Swiss originators, the arthritic hip joint, consisting of the head, neck and upper portion of the shaft of the femur, the thigh bone, are removed and replaced by an artificial hip made of metal. The acetabulum, the hip socket, is reamed out, portions of the bone are removed, holes are made in the socket, and bone cement is placed in the socket. After the bone cement dries and the femur has been properly prepared, the prosthesis is inserted, the range of motion tested, and the incision then closed. This operation is a major procedure but carries very little danger of mortality and for years has proved its worth. At the famed Mayo Clinic, a study of over two thousand such total hip replacements showed that ninety percent of the cases achieved good results.

After several talks with Dr. Houston, Murray Hammond decided in favor of the operation. He obtained a leave of absence from his employers and was admitted to the hospital. A thorough preoperative work-up revealed nothing to contra-indicate the operative procedures, and Dr. Houston assured the family that the risks were minimal and the results excellent. In view of Mr. Hammond's good general health, normal chest X ray, electrocardiogram, blood count and urinalysis, no postoperative difficulties were anticipated.

On the next morning, Murray Hammond was taken to the operating room, where anesthesia was started at 8:25 A.M. by Dr. Reeves, a well-trained, experienced, Board-certified anesthesiologist. The anesthetic procedure took twenty minutes. The patient's blood pressure at the end of that period was 120/75. Surgical preparation was then started, and operating actually began at 8:45 A.M. For fifteen minutes the patient's vital functions were recorded as having followed a normal course. But at 9 A.M., when Dr. Houston was working in the area of the socket of the hip joint, the patient's blood pressure took a sudden drop, and by 9:05 it was recorded as 80/50. It continued to fall to 60/40.

While it is true that the plastic used to prepare the hip socket may sometimes cause a precipitous fall in blood pressure, the pressure usually returns to normal promptly. The fact that Mr. Hammond remained in this state of hypotension was a clear indication of trouble. A rare but well-known hazard of the Charnley-Mueller procedure is the possibility that one of the sharp instruments used to prepare the hip socket could penetrate the bone and enter the pelvic cavity to injure one of the large blood vessels.

If a patient's blood pressure falls from 120/75 to 60/40 it is almost always an indication of severe hemorrhage. If no bleeding is evident externally, an experienced orthopedic surgeon would in this operation immediately recognize the likelihood of bleeding within the pelvis from a lacerated blood vessel. Good practice demanded that several things be done at once. First, Dr. Reeves should have informed Dr. Houston of the patient's hypotension so that the operation could be stopped. There should have been no doubt in the minds of the surgeon and the anesthesiologist that this falling blood pressure demanded prompt attention. Next, Dr. Reeves should have taken all measures to restore Mr. Hammond's blood pressure to normal. Yet nowhere on the anesthetic chart was there a mention of anxiety over the patient's condition. As Dr. Reeves tried, and failed, to counteract the hypotension by giving Mr. Hammond three units of packed blood cells, this should surely have indicated to him that the severe and sustained fall in blood pressure was not due to external operative bleeding; that continued hypotension of this nature must have a primary source somewhere. The pouring in of blood which does not raise the blood pressure must surely mean that as fast as it's being put in at one end it is pouring out somewhere else.

As for Dr. Houston's operative notes, despite his obvious carelessness in surgery, they report an apparently straightforward technical procedure and make no reference to the patient's general condition, or indicate that the anesthesiologist alerted him to the unexplained hypotension.

So, in violation of all good surgical principles, Dr. Reeves continued his anesthesia and Dr. Houston continued the operation until its completion two hours later, the pair of them committing negligence and carelessness of the worst order.

Mr. Hammond was brought to the recovery room at 11:35 A.M. This highly significant note was recorded upon his admission: "Received in recovery room, condition poor, respirations rapid, lips cyanotic, no blood pressure. Patient is awake." This is the description of a patient who is in extreme shock, in this instance hemorrhagic shock. Yet Dr. Houston, in a brief visit to the recovery room, made the astonishing observation that the patient "looked good," and left to go to another operating room and another case.

Mr. Hammond's serious condition seems to have been ignored on the basis of his being awake and talking. It is well known that patients bleeding to death can remain awake and talking until shortly before death occurs. Further evidence that the urgency of the situation was not appreciated was the failure to give any more blood until 1 P.M. Even then no attempt was made to transfuse this blood rapidly; instead it was allowed to run in over the course of one and a half hours. Nor was it good judgment to transfuse packed cells rather than whole blood, but the main point is that the patient still was not being given enough blood in either form.

Finally, at 2:30 P.M. when Dr. Houston returned to the recovery room he called in a general and vascular surgeon, Dr. Moore, to see Mr. Hammond. Dr. Moore noted that the patient's right thigh and leg were cold and that there were no pulses present in the leg, and upon removing the dressings he saw a large mass in the lower right abdomen. He inserted a needle, withdrew blood and promptly took the patient to the operating room with a diagnosis of massive hemorrhage. Upon opening Mr. Hammond's abdomen Dr. Moore found a large, almost complete laceration of the artery which lies behind the hip joint and supplies blood to the entire lower extremity. Surrounding this laceration were almost three quarts of blood. Dr. Moore repaired the artery, using a plastic graft to restore continuity of the blood flow to the lower extremity, and gave the patient multiple transfusions.

The next day, Mr. Hammond had an episode of respiratory arrest, secondary to the trauma of two operative procedures, prolonged shock, massive hemorrhage and inadequate blood replacement. His blood count at this time, in spite of Dr. Moore's transfusions, was less than half of the expected normal. He was treated promptly and vigorously by the resident staff, resuscitated immediately, put on a ventilator and kept in the intensive-care unit.

Two days later Mr. Hammond was in the operating room for a third time, for a tracheostomy. Dr. Moore placed in the patient's trachea a plastic tube which could then be connected to the ventilator. Though Mr. Hammond was treated with care and skill in the intensive-care unit, he showed acute and progressive kidney failure. This was a direct result of his blood loss and prolonged shock during the first operative procedure. As Mr. Hammond now needed hemodialysis, a method of running the blood through a machine which removes the waste ordinarily taken care of by the kidneys, it was decided to transfer him to a neighboring teaching hospital where he would be under the care of a kidney expert.

The attention given Mr. Hammond by this nephrologist, and the hospital, was excellent. He had a number of transfusions, daily dialysis and innumerable blood studies. But in spite of these heroic efforts, Murray Hammond developed a fungal type of septicemia and died after some weeks of treatment. Since Drs. Reeves and Houston refused to admit any negligence, and the insurance company refused the widow an adequate settlement, the case would be coming to trial.

The next afternoon, before my meeting with Mrs. Hammond, I looked through her deposition again, once more appalled at how uninformed the doctors had kept her about Mr. Hammond's deteriorating condition in the hospital. I also got the strong impression of a retiring woman whose life had revolved around her husband and children. There was something almost poignant in the simplicity of her statements about their family life.

Q. During the course of your marriage, were you and your husband ever separated?

A. No, sir.

Q. Of that marriage, how many children were born?

A. We had two.

Q. Was this arthritis that Mr. Hammond had disabling so that he was prevented from doing chores around the house?

A. Well, we did his chores because we figured he went to work and made us a living—

Q. How did he spend his free time?

A. Watching television and listening to a little police radio.

Q. On the average, how much money would he bring home in his paycheck? Mrs. Hammond, if you would like to stop any time, please let me know. I know this is difficult for you.

A. I just can't remember all the figures.

Q. Who would pay, for instance, for pressing of his suits?

A. I did that.

Q. You did that out of your household budget?

A. I did that myself with my iron.

Q. Why after 1973 would you not take vacations?

A. Well, we had bought the larger house and the development we lived in had a swimming pool and we had the big grounds outside and we didn't need to go away. We enjoyed each other's company. My husband and I and the two children, we stuck together . . . We had just about everything we needed right out at our home there. We were happy, we didn't need fancy clothes.

Q. Did you go with your husband on any of his appointments with Dr. Houston?

A. Most all of them.

Q. Can you tell me in a general way what went on when you and your husband would visit Dr. Houston?

A. My husband would undress, Dr. Houston would examine him, bend the leg, the hip.

Q. You would go in the examining room?

A. Yes, sir.

Q. Why would you do that?

A. He was mine and I wanted to see what was going on and know what attention he needed.

Edna Hammond was waiting for me on the side veranda of her sister's two-family house.

"It was real nice of you to come here, Dr. Chodoff." She looked much as I had imagined, a small thin woman with short brown hair heavily streaked with gray. Though her face showed signs of stress, it was easy to find in her neat features and round blue eyes traces of the pretty girl she had once been.

"Please sit down," she gestured, awkward as that girl, to one of the porch lounges. "There's some iced tea, if you'd like. My sister made it before she went out. She had to go downtown to pick up her husband, but she hopes to meet you when they're back."

As though she'd delivered a memorized speech, as well it might have been, Mrs. Hammond sat down and waited for me to speak. I was reluctant to start talking about the case until she felt more at ease. The way she sat forward in her chair looking at me so apprehensively made me very aware of the hospital lounges she'd waited in, the doctors she'd listened to, as she watched her husband change from a healthy man with an arthritic condition to a dying patient. I said the iced tea sounded good, and then I made some small talk about the weather, and I asked if her children were with her.

"No, Jimmy's in school and Marion, she's older, you know, nearly eighteen now—" she smiled for the first time—"though I can hardly believe it. She's looking after him. I don't much like leaving them—not just now . . ." Her voice drifted off and her smile with it.

"I understand, at least a little," I ventured, "what you've been through, Mrs. Hammond. It was a tragic thing to have happened."

She nodded, her eyes lowered. "Yes. To us anyway that's what it is—a tragedy. That's why we can't understand the trouble Mr. Frommer's having to find another surgeon like you who'll go to court and tell the truth about what happened." She looked directly at me, her blue eyes filled with a kind of outraged pain, a look I had become all too familiar with.

"I mean it just isn't right. I told Mr. Frommer he's got to keep looking. There's got to be somebody willing to stand up against Dr. Houston and Dr. Reeves. I'm just not going to let them get away with their lying. They killed Murray, and that's the truth." She spoke in a rush, not so much with anger, a better thing perhaps had it been, but with a bewildered resolution.

"I'm sorry—talking like this. I mean I know there are a lot of good doctors who've dedicated their lives and everything—" She broke off with an uneasy glance at me.

"It's all right, my dear." I put down my glass, wishing I knew how to reassure her. "It's really all right. I'm on your side, you know."

"I do, and I'm real grateful to you. I guess that's why I wanted to see you."

"I think if you can, Mrs. Hammond, you should try to relax about the case. Mr. Frommer is an excellent lawyer, and I'm sure he's going to find another expert witness for you. There's no way any conscientious surgeon can review those files and deny the negligence of the doctors."

Mrs. Hammond kept twisting her handkerchief and smoothing it out again, and I didn't honestly know whether I was consoling her, as I hoped, or only upsetting her more.

"We just thought the world of him," she murmured. "Dr. Houston, I mean. It's still so hard for me to understand how it happened. And when it *did* happen, how he could have acted so casual to us."

I hesitated before answering. "I guess people don't always act the way they might be feeling. You know, Mrs. Hammond, I come from a family of doctors. My father was a good old-fashioned family doctor, my son's a pediatrician, one brother of mine is a psychiatrist, the other's an anesthesiologist. So I really mean it when I say I have a great love for medicine. I think most doctors are honest, decent men. But, well, sometimes things don't always go the way one wants them to. I'm not excusing Dr. Houston in any way, believe me. It wouldn't be possible. I'm only trying to explain that there are times when I think it's the system at fault as much as the individual. Doctors are told they should stick together. When things go wrong, well, sometimes they make it a whole lot worse because they weren't ever taught how to deal with it."

Mrs. Hammond frowned. "I know what you're trying to say, Dr. Chodoff. But it seems to me that doctors are grown-up men like anybody else. It doesn't seem right that they should hide and lie for each other like kids might do."

An ambulance passed by, heading toward the hospital, and Mrs. Hammond gave an involuntary shudder at the sound of the siren.

"I agree," I said. "It's a pretty awful sound. A couple of summers ago I had to take one of those damn things, an old ambulance with no air-conditioning, all the way from Hyannisport to Philadelphia."

She gave me a startled look. "You were driving an ambulance?"

I laughed. "No, not so lucky. I wasn't the driver, I was the patient. I'd been on vacation, sailing, and I started getting chest pains and coughing blood. It was a pulmonary embolus, and the next thing I knew they were bringing me back to Philly in an ambulance."

"That must have been awful for you," Mrs. Hammond murmured, still with a faint look of surprise. I suppose it was at the thought that a doctor could do anything as human as get sick.

"Well, it taught me a little about being a patient. Can't say I liked it much, either. It was the worst trip I ever had. We got caught in one traffic jam for almost an hour. It was near a gas station and a small luncheonette, and finally I just got out of the ambulance and went to the men's room in the gas station. Then I went to the luncheonette and had a hamburger. You should have seen the people in all the cars watching a patient get out of an ambulance, go to the gas station, then to a café and then get back into the ambulance."

Mrs. Hammond's smile was more relaxed, and I told her I'd be interested in hearing just what did happen to her husband if she felt she could talk about it.

"I don't know. I guess the worst thing was that I really trusted Dr.

Houston." She paused. "I felt that with him taking care of Murray at Central everything would be all right. I mean it's not like we didn't really know him. And him us. We weren't new patients or anything. I was the first one that ever went to him, with my husband's aunt when she broke her arm."

"Did the doctor explain the procedure to you before he operated on Mr. Hammond?"

"No, but he told us what would happen after the operation. That Murray would be in the hospital three to four weeks, and that he'd have him walking with a cane by the time I brought him home. That was the last time I talked to Dr. Houston until after the operation. I guess it's what hurts the most, that he didn't right away tell me what really happened to Murray. I know what a busy doctor he is, but still—I mean my husband was in a critical condition. Now, why didn't he tell me that?"

It was a tremulous question, holding more perplexity than resentment. I shook my head. "I don't know, Mrs. Hammond. I wish I did. It just seems that sometimes families are treated as negligently as the patient."

"It's true, I'm not a professional woman but I'd have understood what he was telling me." Mrs. Hammond sat up straighter, a proud little gesture of hers. "I've learned a lot since Murray died. I mean he always took care of most everything. But I kept asking questions until I really found out what happened.

"That first day all Dr. Houston ever told me was that he didn't know what happened. He kind of explained there was a little artery that was pinched and as it opened my husband's blood pressure would go down and as it sealed the blood pressure would come up. He said he didn't know what happened, because during the operation everything was fine, all vital signs were stable, even to the new hip which fit right into place without any problems whatsoever. After the surgery when he was finished with my husband, he took him to the recovery room and prescribed antibiotics and went back into surgery with another patient.

"Well, when the recovery room notified him that Murray's blood pressure had dropped, he asked them to get in touch with Dr. Moore. Then he told me Dr. Moore was going to take Murray back into surgery and repair the artery. When I asked if I could see him before they took him back in, he said they already had him back in. And he left. He had to take another patient into surgery and I didn't see him again until that night." Mrs. Hammond stopped with an apologetic glance at me. "I'm sorry. It's funny, I never was much of a talker—"

"No, it's fine. You go ahead." I wished for her sake she didn't have to relive those scenes, but perhaps this would serve as some sort of exorcism.

"Well, that night, about eight o'clock, he came into the room where they'd had Murray before the operation. He came in very tired and flopped into the chair, and said he'd just got finished. Then he told me again about this little artery being pinched. 'But Murray's going to be all right,' he said, 'Dr. Moore repaired the artery.'

"That was all until the next night." She closed her eyes briefly, as though now trying to shut out the memory. "That was one of the worst days. I had been at the hospital since ten o'clock that morning, and they kept me waiting on the tenth floor. They kept saying they were going to move Murray to the eleventh floor, to intensive care, and when they got him over there I could see him. I was just shoved around all day. My daughter brought Jimmy over when he got out of school, and we just sat there waiting, the three of us.

"Finally, I saw Dr. Houston and he said that Murray was having difficulty with his kidneys—'One has shut down.' I asked if he needed a special nurse. Dr. Houston said, 'No, he's in intensive care.' Then he went to check on him and left the hospital, I guess. I don't know. I didn't see him again."

We were both silent for a while, watching the children play ball in the next yard. I thought perhaps the memories were becoming too painful for Mrs. Hammond, but after a few moments she continued.

"I was so sure my husband was going to be all right. But then the next time I saw Dr. Houston, he was in his operating clothes and he just stuck his head in the door of the room where I was waiting and told me they were contemplating removing Murray to General

Hospital. I told him I didn't like General and he said I had no choice, and he left."

"He didn't explain why he wanted to transfer Mr. Hammond?"

She shook her head. "No. You know, I had always considered Dr. Houston like a friend. I remember the night of the operation, I'd sympathized with him because he'd looked so tired and worn out. I felt close to him. Then the next day when I asked him how the hip was doing, he said, excuse the expression," she murmured apologetically, "'be damned the hip—I'm worried about saving that man's life.' Well, I was pretty shocked hearing it like that, but I told him not to worry because my Murray was a good fighter. I told him he should go home and say a prayer and everything would be all right. I didn't really know what was happening, how bad my husband was, but I had tried to sympathize with that man."

One towheaded youngster missed the ball, and it came rolling up to the porch. Mrs. Hammond went and got it and, with perfect aim, pitched it back to the boy.

"Nice throw," I said with an appreciative nod.

She smiled. "You said you had children, Doctor?"

"Yes, I have a son and a daughter too. Both grown-up, of course."

"Well, I think maybe you'll understand why I had to do this—sue for malpractice, I mean. People seem really surprised at me. Even my sister, she kept asking me was I sure I wanted to go through with this. 'It's awful, poor Murray gone like that,' she'd say, 'but do you really want to go dragging it into court? It just isn't like you, Edna.' Well, that's what everyone thinks."

Mrs. Hammond made that assertive little movement of hers, sitting up straighter. "I guess nobody knows what they really can be like until the time comes when they have to be that way. The reason I'm going to go through with it is, well, there are two of them— Jimmy and Marion. Oh, I don't mean that they don't have their daddy to support them anymore, though that part's true enough. I've got a home that's mortgaged, and a young boy yet to raise. I didn't have that much education. What jobs I could get now wouldn't be very good-paying jobs. I kind of lost everything with Murray. But that's not what decided me. It was the way Dr. Houston and Dr. Reeves just brushed the whole thing off—like it was of no importance, Murray's dying. And covering it up with lies. There wasn't any dignity to it. I didn't want the father of my children to go like that.

"It was an awful ordeal for us to sit in that hospital ten to twelve hours a day and see their dad suffer. Dr. Houston never contacted me, never showed no concern to me over my husband. I had to find out what happened and why it happened. The night after the operation Jimmy was there at the hospital with Marion and me. You try to cover up, try not to admit there's something wrong, to a thirteen-year-old boy. But he knew something had happened. He told me he wished if Dr. Houston was slipping he would have slipped before he took his daddy in there. When things got worse, Jimmy insisted on being at the hospital all the time like his sister and me. One night after we got home he stood by his father's chair and he broke down and cried. He just asked God not to take his daddy away because Dr. Houston made a mistake."

Mrs. Hammond paused for a long moment.

"Then after Murray died and was buried my son kept asking me to see if there wasn't something we could find out. He said he felt like it was all wrong. I remember we were sitting there watching television, and on the television they were talking about life, and a thirteen-year-old boy looked at me. 'Mom, what's left in life,' he said, 'when you don't have a father?'

"I went to bed and I thought it over. I made up my mind I'd have to try to see what had happened. I have to try to clear this boy's mind up." Mrs. Hammond did not cry, although I think we were both afraid she was finally going to.

"Listen to me, going on like this, I'm sorry, Dr. Chodoff. It really helped, though, talking. Most people, unless something like this happens to them, they can't understand. I mean when a man's got some awful sickness and he's in the hospital dying, well, that's God's will. But when it's like what happened to Murray and the doctors don't want to talk to you about it and it's all hush-up and lies, well, a man's death just doesn't have any dignity to it." She paused. "Maybe that's not exactly the word I mean."

I nodded, deeply touched. "I think it is, Mrs. Hammond, exactly the word."

A month or so after our meeting I received a note from Edna Hammond thanking me for my "house call" and telling me that a famous English orthopedic surgeon was going to come from London to testify for her. Not long after this, Edward Frommer called to say that a date had finally been set for the trial.

"I hear you had to go all the way to England to find Mrs. Hammond an expert witness."

"True. And they say there's no conspiracy of silence. Half a dozen orthopedic surgeons read the file, they all agreed it was 'shocking,' but only an Englishman was willing to testify. Though as it turns out we were lucky the others refused. You've heard of David Hemley-Meers?"

I had indeed heard of this renowned surgeon. "You are in luck," I told Frommer. "He's an excellent man."

"You know what he said? He said if he hadn't read the medical files himself, he wouldn't have believed it. He said the anesthesiologist's deposition was incredible."

"I'm glad for Edna Hammond. She deserves a break."

"She certainly does. Though, frankly, I'm not all that sanguine. Did I tell you the defense has the city's medical panel testifying?"

"Oh, Lord," I said, my spirit sinking a little, "there'll be an 'impartial' opinion, of course?"

"Of course. Well, right now all we can hope for is a good jury and, for once, maybe some justice."

On the morning of the trial I spoke to Mrs. Hammond for a few moments in the corridor outside the courtroom. Her children were sitting on the bench with her: a daughter who looked as her mother must once have, and young Jimmy, a thin nervous boy with a sad, wary expression. It is not always an easy thing for me to remain unemotional when I'm participating in cases like this. I have to remind myself repeatedly that as an expert witness I am there simply to give testimony about the facts. But I admit that on this particular day, watching the impassive faces of the seven men and five women who made up the jury, catching glimpses of the impeccably dressed defendant doctors with their self-righteous airs, I found it very hard not to be appalled by what had happened to Murray Hammond, and worried about what was going to happen now to his family.

Nothing could excuse or justify the negligence of Dr. Reeves, the anesthesiologist, or Dr. Houston, the orthopedic surgeon, in continuing to operate for two hours on a patient in hemorrhagic shock. Yet, making a travesty of the medical profession and a circus ground of the courtroom, they presented their defense. Or rather, in frequent hasty consultations with their respective lawyers, the defendant doctors tried to pin the blame on each other for Murray Hammond's death.

Dr. Reeves testified in an interesting progression of memory that (1) he didn't remember whether or not he told Dr. Houston of the patient's fall in blood pressure, (2) "probably" he told him and (3) he "thought" he told him.

Dr. Houston claimed, and repeated often, that at no time during the operation did Dr. Reeves inform him of the patient's critical condition. This statement the anesthesiologist vigorously denied.

Dr. Reeves testified that he had given the patient three units of packed red cells, and Dr. Houston testified that the average amount of blood loss during a hip replacement was three pints. Since there was no *external* evidence of excessive blood loss, it should have been quite apparent to both surgeon and anesthesiologist that the sustained and severe low blood pressure was due to *internal* bleeding. Yet each refused to admit that Mr. Hammond had been in hemorrhagic shock, and both continued to deny the testimony of the nephrologist who stated unequivocally that the patient's death was a direct result of the arterial laceration, the hemorrhage, and the untreated shock resulting in acute renal damage.

It took question after question, under cross-examination, before Dr. Houston grudgingly admitted that laceration of the external iliac artery is not part of the Charnley-Mueller operation.

This finally established, Dr. Reeves said he did not think the patient had bled very much from his lacerated artery, because his blood pressure didn't "go down to the floor," an astonishing statement since Mr. Hammond's blood pressure upon entering the recovery room was zero.

In spite of the patient's near-exsanguination, Dr. Reeves stated that he did not think he had lost enough blood to cause kidney damage, and that the arterial laceration and the continued hypotension for close to six hours had nothing to do with his eventual death. Dr. Reeves went further than that. He claimed that his care for Mr. Hammond had not only met the normal standard of care, it had exceeded it.

As for Dr. Houston, despite the recovery-room nurse's classic description of a patient in severe shock, almost moribund, he kept to his original remark that the patient was "looking good" and "there was nothing to indicate that he was in severe difficulty."

I could have cheered when Mr. Hemley-Meers, the eminent British surgeon, took the stand. He was as vehement in his condemnation of the defendant doctors as he had been in the following excerpt from his pretrial report.

> This case presents the unique situation of the orthopaedist continuing a lengthy operation with a patient in shock and the anaesthesiologist blithely continuing anaesthesia without vigorously protesting continuation of a procedure with a patient in the condition of Mr. Hammond.
>
> I think for an anaesthesiologist to say, as Dr. Reeves has said, that he did not remember drawing the attention of the surgeon to the fall in blood pressure because the surgeon was doing his job and Dr. Reeves was doing his, is a flagrant abuse of the responsibility of an anaesthesiologist. I know when I am doing a hip operation, my anaesthesiologist always looks round to see the amount of bleeding. If it is excessive I always inform him. If the blood pressure drops he always informs me. To allow an orthopaedic procedure to go on for two hours with a dropped blood pressure of 60/32 is, in my view, negligence.
>
> This fall in blood pressure was so dramatic and continued for so long, it is very difficult to believe that an anaesthesiologist would not remember having told the surgeon, because I cannot conceive of any surgeon who would persist in surgery on a patient in this situation. Had it been me it would have been my first ambition to get the man out of the theatre as quickly as possible.
>
> To say that the bleeding might have come from the site of the operation because it is a big operation, does not mean

anything. I presume, as in any other hospital, the swabs used in mopping up the blood are hung up and counted, and are there for everybody, including the anaesthesiologist and the surgeon, to see. Most anaesthesiologists if they are terribly worried about blood loss, irrespective of blood pressure, weigh the swabs with a view to accurate blood replacement.

When Mr. Hammond left the theatre I should have thought that all the sources one would consider as a cause for his fall in blood pressure should have been re-evaluated almost every fifteen minutes, including palpation of his abdomen over the site of the iliac artery, and this can be done irrespective of the dressings and also aspirated through a needle inserted in the abdominal cavity, which is a well established way of determining in doubtful cases whether there is any intra-abdominal bleeding.

I am sure if I had been the surgeon involved in this case with a patient at the end of operation with a blood pressure like this, I should have been more concerned and have stayed around with the patient rather than, as the surgeon did in this case, go and leave the elucidation of the problem to the anaesthesiologist and the recovery room staff.

Inasmuch as the operation in question is rather like the procedure originated in England by Professor Charnley, I do not believe that there is any variation between the so-called standard of care in the performance of this procedure. I am quite familiar with the carrying out of this operation in the United States. Under no circumstances would any surgeon anywhere in the world continue an operation with a patient in Mr. Hammond's condition.

Although Edward Frommer had said that this was going to happen, I was nonetheless upset when the defense called a member of the city's medical panel to the stand. Supposedly it is a panel created to investigate malpractice claims in an unbiased fashion, but there was no pretense as to why Dr. Bell was in court: he was there to whitewash his colleagues. His opinion, along with that of the other members of the panel, was that Mr. Hammond's death was due to fungal septicemia, and that the arterial laceration and shock were not the direct causal agent of death. He also made the amazing statement on the witness stand that Dr. Reeves's care of the patient was exemplary, and that even had he known of the hemorrhage the treatment would have been exactly the same.

When I was called to the witness stand, the opening ploy of the defense attorneys was familiar. My credibility was attacked and the usual attempt made to persuade the jury that I was really not a practicing surgeon but only an itinerant professional witness. After these personal assaults were disposed of, the defense attorney asked how long it would have taken me to make the correct diagnosis when Mr. Hammond's blood pressure began its precipitous fall at 9:05 A.M. I answered five to ten minutes. This, of course, was in extreme contrast to the five and a half hours it took the defendant doctors.

I testified that in the absence of any unusual bleeding at the operative site there was the obvious possibility of injury to a vessel within the pelvis. Since the most probable vessel to be injured would be the external iliac, and since this is the artery whose continuation supplies most of the blood to the lower extremity, the femoral pulse in the right thigh would be diminished or absent, color changed and decreased skin temperature apparent.

Therefore, step number one would have been to remove the drapes and examine the leg, feeling for the femoral pulse. The second step would have been to introduce a central venous-pressure catheter through a vein in the neck, arm or upper chest down to the superior vena cava, the huge vein that returns blood to the heart from the upper part of the body. In a situation such as Mr. Hammond's when severe hemorrhage has occurred, the pressure would be markedly decreased. This ascertained, the surgical procedure on the hip would have been stopped and an exploration of the pelvic vessels started.

Q. Now, Doctor, do you have an opinion what effect, if any, the delay in repairing the iliac artery until 2:30 in the afternoon, what causal effect, if any, did such a delay have on Mr. Hammond's death?

A. Yes, I have an opinion.
Q. What is your opinion?
A. I think it was directly responsible for his death.

All the facts had at last been revealed to the patient's family. Now it was up to the jury to decide who had lied, who had spoken the truth.

It was with deep gratification that I heard that a substantial verdict had been brought in for Edna Hammond, the plaintiff.

9

SHORTLY AFTER THE Hammond trial, Dan Haber and I went out to Bloomington, Indiana, for a medical meeting. It was one of Dan's rare trips away from what he calls his "ivory tower lab," and I was pleased to have his company. He, for his part, was convinced that he saved me from turning the first night's dinner into a banquet-room brawl. And for a few moments, as I later admitted to Dan, I did think the scene might well explode into one of those custard-pie-throwing climaxes of the silent films.

"Silent because they were all speechless with rage," Dan pointed out.

"Hardly my fault that they have such short tempers."

"Oh, really?" Dan laughed. "Those waitresses weren't red in the face from steaming lobsters, my friend, it was your language."

The little contretemps at dinner had started with a Boston neurosurgeon applauding a recent article in one of the American College of Surgeons bulletins. Briefly, it had to do with a suggested plan for a surgical advisory service that would provide confidential advice to colleagues accused of malpractice, assist them and their attorneys in evaluating the medical aspects of a case and, as the doctor warmly quoted, "provide moral support to a Fellow at a time when he may well feel fearful, depressed and isolated."

"A very compassionate plan," said a general surgeon sitting across the table from me. "What do you think, Dr. Chodoff?"

156

I suppose the image of Edna Hammond's bewildered grief was still very much with me, for I replied, "It's a fine concept but hardly original. Don't you think it might be just a little bit more compassionate to organize a service for the injured patient, for the family whose breadwinner was killed by negligence?"

Well, that got quite a reaction from the surgeon, who banged his fist down on the table so hard he knocked over his water glass. One word led to another—familiar ones like "traitor" from the surgeon and his friends, nouns more profane than that from me, I fear. By dessert, the row was such that Dan, with great diplomacy and even quicker action, maneuvered me out of the banquet room and into the soothing dimness of the hotel's bar.

"You want a nightcap before you turn in?" he asked.

"Yes, but small. Enough excitement for one night." I shook my head, feeling a sudden weariness. "It's hard to believe that there weren't some doctors in that room who feel the way I do."

"I'm sure there were. Doctors like me," Dan paused, searching for the words, even though they were so familiar to us both, "who feel like you do, who basically agree with you but who happen to think the answers have to come from the right place so that they'll have real meaning, lasting value."

"Oh, please, spare me, Dan. It's the same old story."

"Okay, so traditions don't change overnight. How could they? But that doesn't mean that one of these days the profession won't wake up to some new responsibilities."

"And meanwhile?" I asked, still thinking of the Hammond family. "Sounds to me, old buddy, that our dialogue is back to square one."

Dan shrugged, and gave his half-wistful, half-sardonic smile. "Since when is consistency a crime?"

I did not have to go to out-of-state trials, of course, to learn about the malpractice problem. A local newspaper published a report of eighty deaths in Philadelphia hospitals over the past ten years which the medical examiner's office suggested might involve malpractice. A mortality-survey committee was set up by the Philadelphia County Medical Society, but the findings were not made public.

Some time later a special committee set up by the State Board of Medical Examiners and Licenses again reviewed those eighty cases, and they concluded that fourteen of the deaths were the direct result of medical negligence. Newspaper reporters then discovered that of these fourteen cases only three families had been told the true circumstances of death. In the other eleven cases nothing had been said to the survivors about what had actually gone wrong.

Also on my mind was the recent brush I'd had with two local "knife-happy" surgeons. It's a kind of despair that drives me to use the term, but that minority of dishonest physicians cannot be denied and should not be ignored. A little boy was sent to me with a pain in the abdomen which was not typical of appendicitis. After thorough examination, blood count and observation for a few hours, I decided that the child did not have a surgical abdomen. I told his mother to take him home but keep in touch with me or her family physician if any untoward symptoms developed. Several days later she telephoned me, extremely upset, and accused me of being a disgrace to the medical profession. Why was I berated? She had taken her son from my hospital to another one, where a surgeon had examined the boy and told her that he needed to be operated on immediately. This surgeon had removed the appendix, described it as being so badly inflamed it was about to "burst," and told the mother that in another two hours her little boy would have developed peritonitis and might very well have died.

If this was true, it was the kind of mistake that I have seldom made and I was worried. As I happened to know the pathologist at the other hospital, I called and asked him to give me the report on the boy's appendix. I was not surprised to hear "normal appendix." *Res ipsa loquitor*—The thing speaks for itself.

The other case had to do with a patient I'd known since her childhood. As a little girl she had been brutally assaulted by her brother, and, as a result, she had grown into a neurotic young woman. She came to see me with complaints typical of gallstones, so I sent her to a radiologist for a gall bladder X ray. This was returned, showing an absolutely normal gall bladder. Accordingly I said to her, "Betty, your gall bladder is normal and there is no need for surgery." She insisted that her symptoms were so severe that in spite of the X rays she wanted the operation. I told her we'd wait a few weeks and then repeat the X ray. This was done and a normal gall bladder was demonstrated. Again Betty insisted that she was suffering and wanted her gall bladder removed, and again I refused.

About three weeks later Betty came back to my office and told me that a professor of surgery at one of the large medical-school hospitals in the city had strongly recommended a gall bladder operation. "Now, if he wants to take it out, why don't you?" she demanded. I argued with her to no avail. Finally, in an attempt to keep her away from this unprincipled surgeon, I said, "Betty, I'll make a bargain with you. I'll open your abdomen. I'll look at your gall bladder, and if it is normal I will not remove it. Are you willing to go through this?"

She said, "I am so miserable I will undergo anything."

I took Betty to the hospital, operated on her, found an absolutely normal gall bladder and did nothing. However, I thought I would try some psychology on my unhappy young friend, and when she recovered from the anesthesia I said, "Betty, your gall bladder was normal but there were some adhesions around it. I divided the adhesions and you should be just fine now."

From that day on Betty never had another gall bladder symptom. However, within a few months she developed all the symptoms of a kidney stone. Needless to say, she had no stone, only the need for long-term psychiatric care, which, unfortunately, she could not afford.

It has been suggested by members of the U.S. Department of Health, Education and Welfare that approximately five percent of American doctors are incompetent or unscrupulous. This means there are something like sixteen thousand doctors undeserving of their medical licenses. Yet statistics from the Federation of State Medical Boards show that in the last decade state licensing agencies have revoked fewer than seventy medical licenses a year. And what of the remaining "incompetent or unscrupulous" thousands let loose on an unsuspecting public?

How many, I wonder, are like the infamous Dr. John Nork. A California physician who was an alleged drug addict, he performed unnecessary back operations for over ten years, disabling a total of over fifty persons. Some of his colleagues were aware of his tendency to "make mistakes," but they did nothing about it. Though Dr. Nork's postoperative reports indicated that the patient was making a remarkable recovery, the nurses' notes invariably showed that the patient was in pain and having problems. As the hospital had no way of monitoring the actions of its doctors, the facts of Dr. Nork's incredible practice were not discovered until a trial lawyer, working under the contingency-fee system, had spent months on the investigation.

Another similar menace was a neurosurgeon employed by a large Midwestern university. His incompetence had caused a partial paralysis to one of his patients. Five months before the operation this neurosurgeon had been hospitalized, at his university, for treatment of alcoholism and depression. Two months before the operation he had been hospitalized for attempted suicide. He admitted to being an alcoholic for twenty years; dependent upon mood-altering drugs; bothered by a tremor for the last ten years; that he had not been dry for more than forty-eight hours in the previous four months. Despite this extraordinary history, the university produced five local neurosurgeons who tried to justify not only the actions of the operating neurosurgeon but also the university's actions in maintaining him on their staff.

The evenings that Paula and I spent with the Habers, or with my son Bill and his wife, generally ended up in what Paula called "shop talk." It followed the same circular pattern no matter how often or thorough our discussions. We all agreed there had to be a way for doctors to maintain reasonable insurance rates; that the medical profession desperately needed more effective policing; that disciplinary action must extend beyond the hospital the offending physician is resigning from. What benefit to the patient if the hospital taking action against a doctor does not, as is so often the case, notify other hospitals? Of course, when we stopped to examine the existing system of discipline it would always dampen the hope, Dan's primarily, that this could be the main solution. Hospitals have, at best, limited authority; specialty boards, none; medical societies and professional-standards-review organizations, little. In fact, only the Board of Medical Examiners has total disciplinary authority.

One big recurring question was, Were there no better, quicker means by which a patient could be compensated for injury? We would discuss all sorts of possibilities based on arbitration boards, no-fault insurance or a workmen's compensation law, until Paula would point out that they were probably unconstitutional and, in any case, were unfair to the patient, who would still be required to prove malpractice.

There was no doubt in anybody's mind that a part of the malpractice problem has to do with the deterioration in communication between the patient and the doctor. Since the coming of the era of specialization the warm personal relationship of my father's day has become obsolete. The very notion of pressing charges against a doctor was unthinkable in those days—it would have been analogous to turning in a member of one's own family. Now the patient finds himself dealing with specialists and often an impersonal efficiency that does little to inspire trust and loyalty. Frequently the doctor is too busy to be reached, or to fully explain a patient's condition and the curative procedures involved in his case. For a physician to ignore the needs, and the rights, of a patient is to betray more than his profession, it is to betray humanity itself.

There is also the continuing problem of hospital care. A manual put out by the Joint Commission on the Accreditation of Hospitals states that "there must be assurance that the attainment of accreditation means that a high quality of care is being provided within the hospital." According to the JCAH the staff of each hospital can contribute to this assurance by means of appointing a peer group to evaluate their work on a regular systematic basis. This includes tissue review and autopsy reports, evaluation of pre- and postoperative diagnoses, the indication for surgery and the quality of consultation. In large hospitals such a committee's checking on quality care is far more apt to be efficient and impartial than that of small, nonaccredited hospitals. But even in large hospitals, influence of patient referrals often blunts the edge of deserved criticism.

The particular subject of "tissue committees" came up one night in a discussion with Dan and an old friend of ours, a general surgeon named Irwin Morris. Irwin had been at Jefferson Medical School with us and then had gone out to San Francisco, where he interned and eventually set up a practice. He and his wife had come back on a family visit, and we three had got together for a reunion of sorts. Irwin felt that the tissue committee at his hospital, while far from perfect, probably helped things.

"There are embarrassing situations, naturally. I mean these are people you see every day, some of them socially. And there you are having to quiz the experts. So it stays polite, but I don't really think much goes unnoticed. The committee meets maybe once a month. Can you imagine, twelve of us sitting around discussing cases while the beepers beep and the doctors come and go. Most of the cases are referred by the hospital pathologist. A normal uterus was removed, so the committee asks why."

"I'd like to know the answer to that," I said.

"Well, the last time it was painful periods, drugs didn't help, and the woman had to miss several days of work a month."

"That was an acceptable answer?"

Irwin shrugged. "I don't know that I'd have advised anything quite so drastic as surgery, but it's a question of judgment."

Dan poured us all some more wine. "Who was the surgeon, a famous guy, who said, 'You can teach a chimpanzee to cut and sew but you can't teach him judgment'?"

On this note the conversation took its inevitable turn back to the patient. The strange lack of communication between Mrs. Hammond and Dr. Houston was still troubling me.

"Come on, Dick, it's not all that uncommon," Irwin protested. "That's where we have a real problem. Doctors aren't as close to their patients as they used to be. Everybody's too busy. But, personally, I don't think it's always the doctor who's to blame."

I smiled. "That has a familiar ring to it."

"No, I'm serious. Patients have to ask the questions they want to ask, assert themselves a little, not just accept every damn thing a doctor tells them. Maybe if they stopped treating us like we're omnipotent, we'd stop acting that way. The English have this joke about patient compliance. The doctor says, 'We've scheduled you for a decapitation next Thursday, Mrs. Jones.' And Mrs. Jones says, 'Fine. Thanks so much, Doctor.' "

"A grain of truth there, maybe," I admitted. "But you take

hospital patients. They don't know what's happening to them. They ask the nurse, she says the doctor will explain, and, frankly, a lot of physicians I know damn well don't want to bother. They get almost defensive about talking to patients."

"I agree," Dan said. "How many doctors do you know, Irwin, that you can even accuse of having a bedside manner? They don't linger there that long. Not like Struthers, right, Dick?"

I laughed. "Now, there was the bedside manner *par excellence*. I don't think anybody ever had the patient rapport he did."

"Who was Struthers?" Irwin asked.

"After your time," Dan said. "He was our professor of obstetrics, one of the sweetest guys I've ever known."

"All the interns loved him," I said. "He never gave us hell and he'd always back us up in arguments with the head nurses."

"He was easily the busiest doctor I've ever known," Dan interrupted. "His patients adored him. With good reason, too. Every Sunday morning the intern on the service would meet Dr. Struthers in the lobby, and he always had a huge bouquet of flowers that he'd just bought at the florist's. So he'd say to the intern, 'How many patients do I have today?' And if the answer, for example, was twenty, we'd divide the flowers into twenty smaller bouquets."

"Then came rounds and at each floor he'd ask, 'Now who is on this floor?' And the intern would say, 'Mrs. Smith—Room 1224.' In Struthers would go. 'Dear Mrs. Smith, I was in my garden this morning,' he'd say, 'and I saw these lovely flowers, and I said to myself wouldn't Mrs. Smith love them.' This act would be repeated on each floor, in each room, the only difference being the name. Later in the day, when we made afternoon rounds, we would always be greeted with exclamations of affection for the doctor. 'What a wonderful man to think of me personally, when he's so busy.' And the thing of it is, he always did make some effort."

"Too bad you can't teach compassion," Irwin said.

"I've always thought we should give it a try," I said.

"Good luck to you. It's been my experience that clichés like 'You can't change human nature' survive because they're true."

"Granted. But I'm not talking about changing human nature, only human behavior."

"Hold on," Dan said, always warming to the conversation when it wandered into a more abstract realm. "If a person is incapable of a real emotion you can't instill him with it." He grinned. "Unless you're talking about some kind of transplantation procedure the rest of us don't know about yet."

"The world's already too plastic," Irwin said. "Who needs ersatz compassion?"

"Unfortunately we do," I told him. "You'd be surprised how much even a semblance of sympathy can mean to a patient."

"So what do you prescribe, Doctor?" Dan asked.

"I think we should start at the beginning. Medical students have to be taught differently than we were. A young doctor should learn that his primary responsibility is to his patients, not his colleagues. That a very essential part of taking care of a patient is the psychological factor. And that should extend to the family too."

"In other words," Dan said, "you're saying let's give courses in humanity?"

"Precisely. And there's something else wrong with the doctor–patient relationship. There's no common language."

We went on, in this way, the three of us, until early in the morning, dreaming up the ideal curriculum for our medical students. An enjoyable night, and profitable, if only to ourselves.

Such dreams of a medical utopia were soothing to the spirit, but within a month I was brought back to earth by the harsh reality of the present malpractice situation. My medicolegal work was not always confined to reviewing files and testifying in court. There were also occasions, as in the case of Jennifer Dresden, when I was called upon not just to give an expert surgical opinion but to repair the injured patient.

The most dramatic hours of surgery I ever spent were in trying to undo the damage done Miss Dresden, a twenty-four-year-old dental assistant from New Hampshire who suffered an incredibly bungled abortion. It was an inarguable charge of malpractice; the injury was an accepted fact over which the attorneys for the plaintiff and the defendant would eventually negotiate a settlement. But when I entered the case the prime concern of Stanley Blume, the plaintiff's lawyer, was his client's well-being.

Stanley was an old patient of mine as well as a friend. "I'm going to put it right on the line, Dick," he said when he first telephoned about Jennifer. "I don't know whether she can be fixed up. The opinion here is that she can't, but it seems too damn hard if that girl has to go through life with a colostomy. My own feeling is that if there's any surgeon who can help her it's you."

"What happened, Stan?"

"A real horror story." I could hear him lighting his *verboten* cigarette. "Jenny's a nice kid, a good girl, and she's been living through a nightmare, pure hell. I'm sure she thinks it's some kind of retribution. Anyway, she got pregnant. The guy, well, it wasn't a good situation and things being the way they were, she went into the hospital for an abortion."

"Suction?"

"Right, and while the gynecologist is doing it he sees something in the suction curette and he isn't sure what it is. So he keeps pulling down on it and pulling down on it. And then finally, too late, he recognizes that what he's got hold of is a segment of the colon. He's ripped it clear away."

"Oh, God. Was anybody else there to help?"

"He called in a surgeon, who did the colostomy. He's the fellow who doubts the bowel can be put back together again. According to this surgeon Jennifer's got a permanent colostomy."

"He could be right, Stan."

"Maybe, but it's your opinion we want. I'm sending on the hospital charts—and the depositions. The liability, of course, is no issue here. Indefensible incompetence. They'll try to bargain over the amount of compensation, but right now I'm not worried about a settlement. It's the girl. She's had a rough year with that colostomy, it's really devastated her. Her father says there's a whole personality change; she won't go anywhere, doesn't want to be with people. See what you can do for her, will you, Dick?"

A week later I received the files and, shortly thereafter, a call from Paul Dresden asking for an appointment to bring his daughter to see me. In reviewing the case I found that the doctors' depositions told basically the same story I had heard from the plaintiff's lawyer. While performing the suction abortion, the gynecologist pulled down a segment of colon. Realizing, finally, what he had done, he called for a surgeon to come to the operating room. The surgical consultant saw that the gynecologist had perforated the patient's uterus, tearing away a large segment of her left colon from its blood supply, and he took immediate action. He removed that torn segment and did a colostomy on the upper end of the colon, closing and dropping the small lower segment. It was not hard to understand his pessimism over any future corrective surgery.

I ought perhaps to have been better prepared for Jennifer from Stanley Blume's descriptions, but adjectives like "nice," "good" and even "devastated" do not convey much over the telephone. A slender girl with large round blue eyes, curly red hair and a crop of freckles, Jennifer had the charming gamine appearance of a grown-up Orphan Annie. But the spunk and animation that clearly belonged on her face were missing. She wore instead an expression of utter misery, a kind of abject humiliation that I wished with all my heart I could help erase.

After I had examined Jennifer, I suggested that she and her father and I talk things over.

"Well, Doctor?" Mr. Dresden said as soon as we were seated in my office. "Do you think you can do anything to help Jennifer?"

I hesitated. "This is what we must discuss."

"Mr. Blume was hopeful that you could—"

I sighed. "Mr. Blume is an excellent lawyer, but as far as medicine goes—"

"Yes, of course, I understand," Mr. Dresden said, with an apprehensive glance at Jennifer. He was a tall, thin middle-aged insurance broker, a divorced father who had been left with three children to bring up. His was the type of rough, furrowed face that showed all emotions, and on it I read not only dismayed concern for Jennifer and a deep supportive love but also that vague hovering guilt many parents have when terrible things befall their children, as though they ought to have taken a firmer hand with fate itself. "Just what is your opinion of the situation, Doctor?" he quietly asked.

"Quite honestly, I don't know what to tell you." I addressed my answer directly to Jennifer. "I want very much to help you, but it would be an extremely difficult procedure to bring the bowel back together. We have an abdomen with multiple dense adhesions, a uterus enlarged to approximately twice its normal size." I made a rough anatomical sketch as I talked, attempting to illustrate my words for the Dresdens. "An abdomen full of massive adhesions can make identification of normal structure nearly impossible. To find the rectal stump under these conditions and then join the upper large bowel to the rectum—well, frankly, I can't even guess at the chance of success."

"But it's the only chance I've got," Jennifer said in a barely audible voice. "I don't think I can live with this thing. I don't want to live if it has to be this way."

"Now, Jenny," Mr. Dresden quickly said, "you can't let yourself think that way. There're thousands of people who lead perfectly happy, normal lives with colostomies. Isn't that right, Doctor?"

"Oh, absolutely," I began.

"No, it's not the same, Daddy," Jennifer said. She had not spoken much until this moment, and now the words came in a desperate blurting. "Most people are older when it happens to them. They already have their husbands, their lives to go on with. But I don't think I can make another life for myself now—not when I'm like I am with this new . . . orifice." She grimaced, her face so pale that the freckles looked raised. "I don't like to be around people anymore. I mean the colostomy—it makes such awful little noises and I never can tell . . . I never know when the bag's just going to fill up." Her voice faltered, barely a whisper now. "And the way it smells—"

"Jennifer," I interrupted firmly, "I never said it would be impossible for me to restore things to normal. I only wanted to explain that there's no guarantee. It's going to be hard, but I think maybe I can do it. I'm willing to try if you are."

For the first time I saw the glimmer of an Orphan Annie spunky smile. "It's a deal."

I admitted Jennifer to the hospital, prepared her for surgery and in a few days took her into the operating room. Though I went in with a certain amount of trepidation, it was even worse than I had imagined. The operation began early in the morning and continued until evening, when finally I closed the patient and went out to talk

167

to Mr. Dresden, who had been waiting for these many hours, fortunately in the care of Mrs. Maxwell.

"Jennifer's going to be all right," I said. "She's going to live a normal life without a colostomy."

Mr. Dresden wept unashamedly, and Mrs. Maxwell, herself vastly relieved, began to cluck at me for "looking quite gray in the face" and insisted on my eating the lunch she had put aside for me some six hours earlier.

Well, I don't doubt I did look a little gray by then. I believe this was probably one of the two or three hardest procedures I'd ever done. Jennifer's abdomen had been a veritable jungle of adhesions, everything matted together and obliterating all anatomical landmarks. After long, tedious dissection I found a segment of dense thickened material low down in the pelvis adherent to the posterior pelvic wall. This proved to be the previously closed and infected rectal stump. The wall of the upper portion of the remaining bowel was so scarred that it could not hold sutures. However, we persisted and eventually did succeed in rejoining the bowel. As a safety measure to promote healing of the newly joined pieces of bowel, a temporary colostomy was done.

When Jennifer came back to her room and heard the news I thought she was going to bolt out of bed, so joyful was her reaction. I explained that to help the healing process she would have to put up with a colostomy for another four weeks, and she just grinned. "Now it will seem like four seconds," she assured me.

Before she left the hospital we closed the temporary colostomy, and Jennifer returned to New Hampshire with her gastrointestinal tract restored. Some six months later there was a three-way conference about the case between me, an "expert" gynecologist and the defense lawyer. As a result of this medical summing-up, Stanley Blume eventually received a satisfactory settlement for his client. But far more important to us all was the news that Jennifer had gone back to work and was again living a perfectly normal life.

10

THE WINTER OF 1980 I remember as being unusually severe.
recall one evening in February when I turned from my desk t
watch the thick pattern of snowflakes in the light of the street lamp:
It was the end of a long day, though there hadn't been enough hou
in it by half. Today I needed what my mother used to call "anoth
set of twelve." Three scheduled operations had been followed by a
emergency, a woman in her late seventies with perforated diverticu
litis and an abdomen full of pus. After that a surgical-staff meetir
and hospital rounds, and only now had I finished with my la
afternoon appointment.

The interoffice phone gave its quiet buzz. "Those anatomic
charts you wanted for Mr. Jameson are here, Doctor."

"Oh, good. Bring them in, please."

Mrs. Maxwell came in with an armload of colored charts aı
diagrams.

"Thanks. You'd better get on home before you're snowed in."

"Is there anything you need before I go?" She hesitated, looki
at me with that discreet blend of concern and disapproval, a lool
knew well. "How much longer do you plan on staying, Doctor?"

"Just a couple of hours or so, Virginia. You go on, I'll be fine.

"Did you remember to take your medicine?"

I sighed. "No. And I don't think a man of seventy-one has to
reminded like a child."

"Nor do I."

"The more you and Paula fuss over nothing, the more apt I am to forget."

Our banter ended, as it usually did, with my good friend winning the round, and I took the anticoagulant that I should not, in fact, be quite so forgetful about. For in the last several years I'd had two more pulmonary emboli, the last rather recent.

"And now will you go home, Mrs. Maxwell?"

She smiled. "Yes, Dr. Chodoff."

I looked over the charts of the upper circulatory system and propped the biggest up against the bookshelf. Here, very clearly, one could see the large artery called the common carotid as it comes up from the heart on each side of the neck. In the upper part of the neck, near the angle of the jaw, it divides into two: the external carotid artery with its many branches conducting blood to the thyroid, the larynx, the face; and the internal carotid artery, which has no branches but goes straight through the neck into the skull, supplying blood to half the brain. It is the complete stoppage of this latter artery that produces hemiplegia, commonly known as a stroke. And that was the precise subject of the lecture I was shortly to deliver to my class of one, a lawyer named Clark Jameson who had come from Kansas to study the pertinent physiological details of the case for which I was to be the expert witness. We had already had two "teaching" sessions; this evening would be the last in preparation for the trial that was coming to court next month.

While I waited for Clark, I took out the plaintiff's medical file and reread the notes of Dr. Paul Miller, the neurosurgeon who first examined Laura Carlson. He described her as an unusually bright young woman, with a successful career and a happy marriage, who visited him because of a curious whistling noise in her left ear. The sound had actually started several years earlier, but until recently Mrs. Carlson had been aware of it only at night when everything was quiet. Now, however, this "interior 'ringing'" sound was beginning to disturb her during the day, the volume increasing when she was excited or angry or, indeed, had any emotional reaction. Her pleasure in music, an interest shared with her husband, was diminished, and, more practically, she now found telephone communication a growing problem. To compensate for the difficulty in hearing herself above the inner sound, she was obliged to raise her speaking voice considerably.

Mrs. Carlson's observations were that the noise stopped at times when she turned her head sharply to the left or if she let it hang down to an exaggerated degree. It was temporarily aggravated or improved with other accidental changes of position, and could be altogether obliterated when she applied pressure against her neck over the carotid region.

Dr. Miller's medical report established Laura Carlson as a healthy, well-developed, well-nourished twenty-seven-year-old black female with quite good hearing, normal facial sensation and symmetrical facial movements. The neurosurgeon detected no bruits over the carotid regions, but did hear a bruit over the left temple in front and just above the left ear. The coordination tests he gave the patient were rapidly and well performed, and she was within the limits of normal in her equilibrium, sensory, motor and reflex examinations.

The conclusion that Dr. Miller drew was that the whistling was possibly due to an anomaly in the circulation of the left external carotid artery; that she should consult a vascular surgeon, who in turn would arrange for a carotid angiogram of the left side to rule out vascular difficulties in both the internal and the external carotid circulation.

Dr. Miller told Mrs. Carlson that as the sound could be stopped by pressure applied to the area of neck where the external carotid artery rises, this might signify an abnormal communication between an artery and a vein leading to the ear area. He explained that such an arteriovenous, or AV, fistula, as it is called, should be easily detected by a carotid angiogram. In this procedure a radio-opaque substance is injected into the carotid artery and the "dye" outlines the internal anatomy of the vessels for the X ray. He then referred Mrs. Carlson to Dr. Robert Ashton, a general and vascular surgeon, with the recommendation that arteriographic studies be carried out and surgery performed *if* a vascular abnormality was found.

Mrs. Carlson accordingly made an appointment with Dr. Ashton, who arranged for her to enter the hospital on November 8,

1977. His admission note read: "This 27-year-old girl has probable small A-V fistula near left ear which produces a constant noise in ear. No strong evidence of trauma. Arteriogram today and surgery tomorrow."

Having already decided in advance that he would operate, the surgeon was not deterred by the fact that his patient's X-ray report was negative. The vessels visualized were normal in course, diameter and configuration. No vascular malformation or displacement was seen.

On November 9, Laura Carlson was taken to the operating room, and at 9:20 A.M. Dr. Ashton began the surgical procedure. His operative notes were as follows:

> Under general anesthesia, an incision was made beneath left lower jaw and carried down through muscle with ligation of the bleeding points. We carefully began to search through the various vessels for evidence of a fistula in this region, identified several veins which did not appear to be grossly abnormal, and slowly and carefully divided these as we progressed deeper into the neck. We then identified what appeared to be the external carotid artery with the branches coming off of it, and one of these branches was quite tortuous, with curves and twists, moderate in size in diameter, and we thought that perhaps it was kinking in this region and was the cause of her fistula. We could not identify a true A-V fistula, and the cause for the ringing in her ear; we felt it could be this vessel or otherwise a fistula that was located within the bone itself and was not amenable to surgery. We then identified these branches and ligated the branch of the external carotid artery, as well as ligating the external carotid artery to reduce the flow to whatever may have been causing the noise. Having performed this, we proceeded to close the wound. The blood loss was minimal and the patient woke without complication.

Would that the doctor's blithe assumption had been true. At 10:35 A.M. Mrs. Carlson went to the recovery room, at 2 P.M. she was brought down to her own room. By 2:35 the nurses' notes had begun to record the persistent headache that heralded her most unusual postoperative course.

By 1 P.M. on the following day, November 10, the patient complained not only of an increasingly painful headache but "a numbness on the left side of the neck including her ear. Stated she still has the 'roaring' noise in her left ear. Dr. Ashton here and changed dressing."

4:30: "Found patient crying from pain of headache in left temple. Medicated for pain. Patient appears uncomfortable and restless."

5:30: "Medication seems not to have helped—patient seems still uncomfortable. Dressing dry—does not appear swollen around left neck area."

7:00: "Husband to visit patient. Patient withdrawn and seems very restless. Patient follows instructions—opens mouth when asked, opens eyes. Pupils equal and reactive. Patient reaches into air as if reaching for something. Patient feels her arm all over. Periods of restlessness and periods of apparent sleep."

7:30: "Patient appears to be less restless—patient seems to respond more to people in room—made some slurred answers to questions—seems aware of people in room. Pupils remain equal and responsive."

9:00: "Medication held due to patient's apparent withdrawal. Dr. Ashton to see. Vital signs remain stable. Patient appears very sleepy—restraints on to keep her in bed. Patient seems very tired."

10:00: "Very restless. Will not speak. Follows simple requests. Grasps at head and ear (left side) but will not verbalize. Most of agitation and activity appears to be on left side. Becomes very restless but if you say her name she'll quiet down. Benadryl 50 given with no apparent relief. Dr. Ashton notified. Chloral hydrate ordered."

Although the nurses had found Laura Carlson's condition at 10 P.M. alarming enough to call Dr. Ashton, he did not come to the hospital. His only response to the patient's ominous neurological symptoms was to order a sedative and transfer her to the intensive-care unit. She was not seen again by Dr. Ashton until 10:45 A.M. on November 11, by which time she was comatose. Dr. Miller, called in for a consultation, felt that the patient must have developed a clot in her internal carotid artery. He advised an immediate reoperation and had Mr. Carlson "alerted to the seriousness of the situation."

The patient was taken to the operating room, and at 12:45 P.M. Dr. Ashton began the second operation, described in part by his following notes.

Mrs. Carlson had undergone exploration of her left neck two days ago at which time we were searching for an A-V fistula and tied off the external carotid artery. She did well for about 30 hours postoperatively with no complaints, was up walking around and ambulatory. Approximately 6 o'clock last night she became aphasic without any localizing neurological signs in regard to the use of her extremities, and had a good grip with both arms. This morning, examination revealed a hemiplegia on the right side. At this time we did not know the exact etiology of this but we certainly had a patient who was in serious condition and we immediately returned her to the operating room. We opened up the old incison under general anesthesia. We found the source of our problem being that we inadvertently tied off both the internal and the external carotid arteries.

In mistakenly having tied off the internal carotid artery, Dr. Ashton interrupted the blood supply to half of Laura Carlson's brain, causing her stroke and loss of speech. In an attempt to correct the situation he removed the tie and the large clot he found within the artery. A graft was placed, and the blood supply was restarted.

In his operative note the surgeon stated that he did not think the patient had suffered much loss of blood supply to the brain from the tie but primarily from the clot, which had extended upward over the thirty-hour period between the two operations. Intended to change the focus of an inexcusable error, this statement served only to condemn Dr. Ashton the more. For had he indeed corrected the situation promptly, the patient would not have suffered as much brain damage.

The day after the second operation, Mrs. Carlson was still semicomatose and restless with purposeless movements of the right leg but none in the right arm. Though she was slightly improved and a bit more alert on the following day, an electroencephalogram showed extensive abnormalities on the right side of the brain. After ten days in the hospital, she was transferred to a center specializing in the care of patients who have had strokes. She remained there for several weeks getting daily physical therapy and speech therapy. Slow improvement continued, and at the end of a year of therapy she was functioning fairly well, although certainly far below her preoperative level. And the whistling noise in her left ear was still present.

The technical errors in this case continued to stagger my imagination. The standards of care to which Laura Carlson was entitled when she went to a qualified surgeon were grossly violated. "Ligation of the offending vessel or similar surgery should undoubtedly be done if such surgery is indicated by the appearance of the angiogram," is what Dr. Miller had recommended. Dr. Ashton's decision to explore the neck although the results of the angiogram were normal, a decision made *before* the test, shows judgment so poor as to verge on negligence.

It is difficult to believe that a certified surgeon could "inadvertently" ligate the internal carotid artery. It is assumed that any surgeon who undertakes to operate deep in a patient's neck has at least some fundamental knowledge of the involved anatomy.

As for Dr. Ashton's postoperative care of Mrs. Carlson, it was completely in violation of accepted standards. She began to show signs of cerebral damage sometime around 6 P.M. on November 10. These signs progressed rapidly and were quite apparent by 7:30 P.M. Dr. Ashton saw her around 9 P.M. but, amazingly, paid no attention to her obvious cerebral difficulties. He should certainly have suspected that thrombosis of the internal carotid artery was taking place, and been quite certain of it when notified of the patient's condition at 10 P.M. To sedate her and send her to the ICU without seeing her was a total breach of medical care.

I looked over some of Dr. Ashton's deposition—a lengthy and agile attempt to sidestep the issues.

Q. Were you the head surgeon with respect to Laura Carlson?

A. Yes, sir, I was.

Q. And when you commenced the surgery, what was it that you intended to do?

A. Mrs. Carlson had a ringing or whistling in her ear on the left side, which clearly by our examinations was due to some form of vascular abnormality, causing the turbulence of blood flow which produces this type of noise. . . . And our intention at the time of surgery was to, if possible, find the exact cause, which I wasn't overly hopeful for because our X rays didn't demonstrate it within the neck, but to divide the blood vessel going to that area to eliminate the blood flow through there which caused the noise.

Q. What examination revealed the vascular abnormality?

A. The examination which verified that presence was auscultation of the neck, which is listening with a stethoscope, in this case to a blood vessel, and it produced an abnormal sound. We term the sound a bruit, which is produced by turbulent blood flow. And this blood vessel is going up past the ear; this noise will be transmitted to the ear and heard as an abnormal noise.

Q. At the time that you saw Laura, did you have in hand Dr. Miller's report?

A. Yes, I did.

Q. Did he give any instructions to you concerning what should or should not be done?

A. I don't know if I can exactly remember. I can say that Dr. Miller had talked to me about Laura before I saw her, I knew a small amount of information, and he then sent the record to me. He did not make a specific recommendation, as I recall, as to what he thought we should do.

Q. Dr. Miller suggests in his report, he says ligation of the offending vessel or similar surgery should undoubtedly be done if such surgery is indicated by the appearance on the angiogram. What he was saying was that if in the converse the angiogram was normal it should not be done?

A. I don't believe you can interpret or infer the negative from a positive statement.

Q. I'm not inferring it. I'm asking if you did?

A. No . . . I would interpret that statement as meaning that he along with myself on my examination felt that there was definitely a vascular abnormality. Then you do the arteriogram. We did not clinically see the deformity that had caused the noise. At that point I did not discuss it with him again as far as I can remember. I did discuss it with the patient, though.

Q. What did you tell her about what she could expect from it, what dangers if any were posed by the surgery?

A. You're asking me to recollect some information that I told a patient two years ago. I can't reconstruct that. She's a young woman undergoing an operation which normally would not have tremendously adverse effects on anybody's respiration or the heart which are the major organs we worry about. So I probably told her there was not a great risk to her. Specifically I don't remember. I told her what we hoped to achieve and what I hoped the results would be. As far as adverse effects, I can't remember specifically. I try to be as honest as I can.

Q. Do you recollect whether or not she was at all concerned about the prospect of surgery?

A. I don't know that she was any more concerned or less than any patient is that undergoes surgery.

Q. To you as a vascular surgeon, was this a particularly complicated surgery compared to the other types of vascular surgery that you do?

A. Well, it's a difficult operation, specifically because we're operating and trying to find a cause of a problem which we can't see directly, and it's difficult in that we're performing an operation to help the patient without a guarantee that we can do it because we can't identify specifically what we're doing, you know, the specific area of the problem, and we're taking this, the slightly perhaps indirect approach.

Q. Now, once you have made an appropriate incision, how do you identify generally the internal and external carotid arteries?

A. We identify them by isolating the area in which they divide and looking at them carefully for the orientation and looking for branches which come off of the external but do not come off of the internal; there are no branches of the internal carotid in the neck, there are branches of the external, and this is perhaps the most reliable method of differentiating between them.

Q. Now, then, with respect to Laura Carlson, is that how you did do it?

A. During the operation on Mrs. Carlson, we approached it from relatively high up under the mandible, and we were looking above this area for an abnormality of the smaller blood vessels initially where the noise may be generated that she was hearing. Not finding a significant abnormality, we identified a vessel in the neck at that level above the area where they bifurcate and we followed that vessel and followed it down along its branches to look for the abnormality. And we saw several branches and one appeared to be abnormal, that turned out to be the internal carotid. But from our viewpoint at that time, it looked to us like just a major branch of the external carotid, it was small, it did not have a normal-size appearance that we would expect of the internal carotid.

Q. Now, you used the word "we" on several occasions. Who is "we?"

A. Well, this is not necessarily "we" in terms of—there is an assistant, and when we talk about surgery we talk about what two people see or whoever else was there. I was the surgeon, so to replace that by "I" would be accurate.

Q. Now, would you expect the incision that you made to have revealed both the internal and external carotid arteries?

A. I think you could view them through that incision, but direct in the manner that I operated I would not expect it. It's a matter of whether you lift up and go downward or whether you go inward, and I felt we were going primarily inward.

Q. Have you in your mind attempted to identify, should you have to perform such a surgery again, what you would do differently the next time than you did with Laura Carlson, if anything?

A. Laura Carlson had an unfortunate result, and obviously I would not want it to happen again.

Q. And has anything occurred to you that would assist you in not having that similar thing happen again; in other words, would you change your procedure?

A. I would make the less cosmetically pleasing incision that would take me down lower in the neck where I could without any question see the common carotid and follow out every single branch of it.

Q. Would you expect an individual who has undergone a surgery which Laura Carlson did to have headaches in the recovery room?

A. If the only complaint that she had was headache, I would not be particularly alarmed by it.

Q. Now, when you go to see a patient where, for example, she apparently did evidence complaints of a severe headache, would you review the nurses' notes?

A. I probably would talk to the nurse. I review nurses' notes frequently. But with an individual patient, I probably would talk directly to the nurse involved. When I saw Laura that evening she had a headache, which is just in my memory the main reason I went to see her. What else I was told I don't recall. And when I examined her I did not find a localized symptomatology. She could move her arms and legs and squeeze your hands and move her feet and talk understandably. She was drowsy, which again is a somewhat diffuse symptom.

Q. Did you identify anything that you considered to be unusual about her speech at the time that you saw her?

A. When I was sure she was aroused, she could talk quite plainly. She wanted to sleep, she was drowsy, and she, as some people are when they are very drowsy, their speech may be slurred. But that cleared when she was awake and could talk.

Q. Let's trot on with the nurses' notes . . . "Will not speak.

179

Follows simple requests. Grasps at head and ear (left side) but will not verbalize. Most of agitation and activity appears to be on left side. Becomes very restless but if say her name will quiet down." We are now opposite the 10 P.M. entry. "Dr. Ashton notified. Chloral Hydrate ordered."

Do you recall being notified sometime after the 10 P.M.—

A. I can't specifically recall that, which isn't—I know my thoughts about it. I had seen Laura earlier in the evening and at that time could not identify, as I say, a localizing sign. One of my impressions was that she might have been a little bit hysterical. She was a rather excitable girl, she had had surgery, she had the headache, and I thought perhaps with the medication she was responding a little bit hysterically, perhaps not personalitywise, but maybe the medication was having that effect on her. Some people, they will hallucinate under pain medication.

Q. Is it your habit to send people with a condition that you felt was generally simply an hysterical reaction, is it your habit to send them to intensive care?

A. I can't answer directly on a question—I'd like to apply what you are asking to Mrs. Carlson. I obviously was concerned about her.

Q. Now, when you ordered Mrs. Carlson moved to intensive care, are there any instructions that you give about being notified about further progress or changes in any conditions?

A. It varies on the individual. You may write a specific order, "I want to know when such and such occurs." Frequently—and understanding these are specially-trained nurses, they contact you fairly often if there is something that I requested them to, which may not be in writing, or for something that would be unexpected associated with the patient's illness, I would expect them to notify me.

Q. Now, the entries that are in the Intensive Care Nurses' Notes starting at 11:15 P.M., and the next entry being 1 o'clock—so apparently that would be the period between 11:15 and 1—are "27-year-old black female admitted to ICU 4 from Surgery West. Does not respond verbally. Restless at intervals. Thrashing about in bed. Moves extremities on left side only . . ." Do those—and not necessarily with the benefit of hindsight, but if that information had been communicated to you, would that then have seemed to be evidence of localizing signs?

A. Obviously.

Q. Well, how did you come to know that Laura Carlson was unconscious—did someone advise you of that, or did you simply see it when you came in the following day?

A. . . . It was distressing. . . . I don't remember . . . if I came in to see her or if they called me. Obviously at the time I saw her it was somewhere in the midmorning or earlier morning, which would be the routine time to be in the hospital, and she was unconscious, that's my recollection of the events.

Q. And at that point in time, what did you do?

A. I called Dr. Miller and I called one of the radiologists to help me do an examination which they had the equipment for, and we determined that she had a blocked carotid artery, and I took her back to surgery. I did not know obviously at that time that we tied off the internal carotid artery, it wasn't the foremost thought in my mind, and until that point, you know, when she clearly had a stroke.

Q. Now, knowing Laura Carlson's physical condition generally, her age and her makeup and her well-being, is there any period of time during which when those localizing signs commenced manifesting themselves that you could have surgically intervened and averted a total hemiparesis?

A. I don't know that there is an answer specifically, trying to be honest. An individual patient has to be their own control as far as determining something like this, and how you have a patient be their own control and also be the experimental resource for your information. But the amount of anoxia that the brain suffers is going to be the determining factor in their recovery, and how long it occurs before you correct it, whether correcting it makes a difference is not known. We corrected it—I'm not positive that that made a difference. We hope it makes a difference. But there's no way to prove scientifically that it did, or that doing nothing would have made any difference.

Q. Following her return from the second surgery, I think you did indicate that Laura was still unconscious initially, is that right?

A. Yes, I did answer such.

Q. I don't know what her next state was—what did you observe about her that indicated some improvement from being totally unconscious?

A. The day following surgery, November 12, I said the patient showed some improvement. She seemed to be awake in terms of where she could open her eyes and understand what we would say to her. She was able to move her right leg some. So she was at least no longer unconscious.

Q. The next entry you have, which I take it would be your next recollection, is what on her condition?

A. She could follow verbal commands, meaning if you asked her to move say her left hand or open her mouth or do something specific, she could do it, which is a general evaluation of her mental status, now that she was waking up quite readily from the coma that she had been in. That the 13th.

On the 14th my note says that her mental alertness was near normal. She could function the left side very well. She had good strength at this time in her right foot and toes. She still could not talk and she still had severe paralysis of the right arm.

Q. Now, would you elaborate a little bit on her mental alertness being near normal, what did you mean by that and how did you determine that?

A. Well, this girl or any individual who has had a cerebral vascular accident who can't speak because of the injury, you have to gauge their alertness by how they respond to specific requests, such as using the good arm, say, to reach out, hold your hand, squeeze, hold up so many fingers, which would give recognition that she could, you know, recognize how many fingers she had. Her thought processes were working relatively well.

Q. The next entry is dated what, and what does it say?

A. Well, the next one is the 17th. Dr. Miller says she is phonating, which is making sounds with her mouth, not exactly words. She is making sounds, or be able to make sounds as she wants to. For the exact ability she had at that time, she was being evaluated at our Stroke Unit, where she had been transferred.

Q. Now, there is a discharge summary which you prepared. Now when you say she was completely able to take care of herself, do we have a patient who when leaving is normal in all respects with the exception of a speech deficit?

A. No, that does not mean that.

Q. Okay, tell me how she was when she left.

A. If she lived alone she could do everything that would be needed to get by, she could walk without assistance—in fact, I believe she could walk without any problem, period, at that stage. She had use of her arms to the point where she could handle things, she could do housekeeping work, she could do cooking. It does not mean that it's totally normal, because as is evidenced in further notes, it isn't totally normal at that stage but it's functional. She was able to have full control of her bladder, her bowels and do the things that you and I do normally to get by. Perhaps not as readily at that time, but still take care of herself. It does not mean a normal individual in every respect.

Q. It's my understanding that following the first surgery and the immediate postoperative care that no further billings were rendered to Mrs. Carlson for any services; do you have any idea why, or who paid them or what happened to them?

A. I charged Mrs. Carlson for the initial operation. The postoperative care of any operation is included in the charge for an operation whether it's minimal or prolonged and complicated care. The cost of surgery is not just the operation, it's the total care for the patient. The second operation on Mrs. Carlson was a complication of the first one, and I can't say what everybody does, but I very infrequently, if I feel it's a direct complication, not something additional, do not charge to go back and to correct a problem which would help the patient.

Q. Now, in addition to that, however, there are separate charges for the hospital care that a patient has while in the hospital.

A. Yes.

Q. And apparently Mrs. Carlson was not charged for those either.

A. I have no knowledge of that.

I was still studying the defendant doctor's deposition when Laura Carlson's attorney finally got to my office for our meeting.

"Sorry I'm so late," he said, taking off his coat. "Between the traffic and the snow . . ." He shook his head and smiled. A fair-complexioned man with black hair and a slight frame, Clark Jameson has an unprepossessing appearance that is as deceiving as his mild voice.

"No problem. I was just looking over Ashton's deposition again. His evasions are incredible. He says the first indication of a stroke was the 11 P.M. ICU notes, and they're almost exactly the same observations the nurses made when they called him at 10 o'clock, for God's sake. Bad enough that he didn't go to the hospital right then, but I'm damned if I understand how that girl could be lying there in ICU, comatose, mind you, until he came by on his rounds in the middle of the next morning. It's another of those damned hospital mysteries. ICU didn't know she was unconscious until he got there? Or they didn't notify him? Or again he hadn't responded? A charming bunch of suppositions." I got up to shake his hand, a little sheepishly. "Hello, Clark, how are you? Didn't mean to greet you with a tirade."

He laughed. "Pleasure's mine. This isn't the first time I've gotten that reaction from a doctor." The intensity of his dark eyes betrayed his casual manner. "The difference is you've been the only one who's agreed to say it in court. And if it weren't for Michael, " he said, naming our mutual lawyer friend, "I'd still be without an

184

expert witness. And we're talking about a big city, a big hospital, big men, and not one of them willing to testify for the girl. Oh, they all condemned Ashton's behavior. Right down the line, operating when there was no need, not coming to the hospital when the nurses called. Yet invite these doctors to air their opinions in court and you get a million excuses." Clark delivered this speech without rancor. Basically an observer, he tends to speak as though he's making some sort of off-the-record commentary on the idiosyncracies of the human race. "Well, let's get on with it, shall we?" he said.

"Right. I've got some material here that might be useful to you, and I want you to go over my deposition and tell me where I need to clarify my medicalese for the jury."

We went over various points of the case until I realized it was nearly nine o'clock and suggested that we break for dinner.

"Good idea," Clark said. "Never thought I'd say such a thing about a hospital cafeteria. Goes to show you what surprises life holds for us all."

That meal we shared in a quiet corner of the cafeteria was really my first introduction to the plaintiff.

"She worked in a brokerage firm, you know," Clark said.

"No, I didn't."

"Oh, yes, an extremely intelligent girl. And absolutely gorgeous."

"I didn't know that either."

"Thought I mentioned all this when we talked on the phone. She comes from a very successful, very well-off black family. Father makes industrial films. It's what you might call a three-star tragedy. Laura had everything—beauty, brains, career, love." He shook his head, adding softly, "And a whistling in her ear. Odd, isn't it, the games fate plays? I mean the girl tries to get rid of this little nuisance and she ends up losing everything but *it*."

"How much brain damage do you think there actually was, Clark?"

"Oh—considerable. She gets around, yes, but this was a powerhouse young lady and she's very slowed down. The facial paralysis is not too disfiguring, but speech is a problem. She's got a bright husband, an architect, who obviously loves her and tries to help, but it's a difficult situation. She was never a dependent type, I gather from her mother. She was one of those kids—an overachiever. I really believe she thought she could come all the way back. Now she still works at her therapy, but she gets discouraged. The mother, on the other hand, is undiscourageable. Is that a word?"

"It is now. What does the mother do?"

"Runs a posh interior-decorating business. She's a very classy lady. Claire Glynn's her name. A beautiful woman and a dynamo. I imagine that's where Laura got her brains and drive."

"What about the brokerage firm? Has Laura considered going back?"

"Constantly. Not a chance, though. She couldn't possibly handle it. I got a deposition from the head of the firm. He'd love to have her back, she was his assistant. Absolutely tops, he said. The customers loved her. According to him, Laura could handle six calls at once, work the quote machine and never take her eyes off the ticker screen. You read the therapists' reports, Dick?"

"Yes, quite protective of Ashton, I thought."

"Well, everybody is. The tactics in a case like this are always the same. 'Laura's not so bad for a stroke patient. Quite good, in fact.' "

"Nobody mentioning the fact that she didn't come to the hospital as a stroke patient, naturally."

"Naturally." Clark shook his head. "Laura's boss said when he first talked to her she sounded like she'd just got off a boat from the Orient. That's a quote. I said, 'You mean her speech was different in some way?' 'Oh, yes,' he said, 'wild!' Poor kid. That's what I mean about fate. Who'd have thought anything as innocuous as a ringing in the ear could lead to losing so damn much?"

"Well, I guess that's what this is all about, isn't it?" I said. "Trying to help her win some of it back."

Three weeks later I flew out to Kansas for Laura Carlson's trial. I'd been thinking a great deal about her case—"brooding" would perhaps be a more accurate word. After our meeting in Philadelphia, Clark and I had several more long-distance conferences, and even on the flight out there I was still preparing myself for court by studying the depositions of the therapists who worked with Laura.

It seemed to me that the hospital's physical therapist had made an undisguised effort to gloss over Laura's stroke, much in the manner of Dr. Ashton:

Q. Now, with respect to coordination of the right hand, do you have any notes or recollection that tell us anything about whether or not there was an improvement last time you saw Laura?

A. As far as handwriting is concerned, this takes a certain amount of coordination and dexterity . . . As far as using the right hand to help her dress and groom, yes, she could use it for that.

Q. How about activities such as typing, this sort of thing?

A. I couldn't answer that. I know that she could pick up small objects with the right hand. As far as dexterity in typing, I don't know that.

Q. Now, when she left could you as a physical therapist determine whether or not looking at her she was just another normal person or did she remain having problems which you could find were related to her previous stroke?

A. Boy, that's a loaded question. Without seeing the individual before when she apparently was normal and afterwards, it would be difficult to judge. I think to see her walking down the hall, if she was in a crowd, you would assume, assume, gentlemen, that she was normal. But upon examination of her right extremities you would find some weakness, I am sure.

Q. When we are talking about weakness, she had weakness in her right hand. She also had weakness in the other extremities of her right side, is that correct?

A. Yes, she did. But the right lower extremity improved so rapidly it was less affected initially than— The major problem was in the right hand.

Q. Now, when you were talking about her ability to communicate to you, you said that she could understand commands and she could make her wants and needs clear to you?

A. Yes.

Q. Again, it isn't intended to be a loaded question in any way, but I know, for example, the monkey Washa in the tests they had developed could also make her wants and needs known and follow commands. The question that I am wondering about, is that the person who left you, as far as communicating to you, was to all intents and purposes a normal person; in other words, when she spoke to you and made her wants and needs known, was that speech as clear as yours or mine?

A. I really couldn't say—that is not my expertise per se—if she had normal speech. I don't have the experience to really test how her abstract reasoning would be and how she could communicate solutions to abstract problems. Just on the surface, she seemed to communicate her needs, seemed to understand verbal communication, and I really don't firmly recollect if I thought she had trouble with speech at the time of discharge. She may have had trouble, but I haven't got it documented and that isn't my province to judge those things per se.

The speech pathologist who worked with Mrs. Carlson gave, it seemed to me, a more honest evaluation in her deposition.

Q. The first symptom that you described was expressive aphasia.

A. Yes. There is receptive aphasia also. Expressive aphasia is a problem in the ability to express yourself. These can be very severe, not be able to think of the words that you need to speak, not be able to put words together for coherent communication, inability to write, because this again is an expressive modality, or inability to make expressions.

Q. You say her major presenting problem was the slurred speech?

A. Yes, that is what I worked with first.

Q. The third one, that was subtle language problems. What would that involve?

A. That would involve using completely precise words for what she would be trying to say.

Q. Could you give me an example of that?

A. Well, Laura is a bright intelligent person and if she were perhaps trying to describe something in detail, something like a painting, she might not be able to get the exact word for a color. She might call it blue instead of turquoise.

Q. During the time that you worked with Laura, how would you characterize her willingness to work with you and her efforts to improve her condition?

A. She was always extremely cooperative, very concerned about her speech. I think at times she got discouraged. She would really work hard at things and still was having some problems.

Q. At the time that she was discharged, if you would give us as complete a picture as you recall both from your notes and recollection as to what Laura's status was.

A. Well, when she talked she certainly could be understood, but her speech was slurred at times and there were certain sound combinations that it was difficult for her to make. She was also talking about wanting to go back to work but feeling that she couldn't do the kinds of things that she had done before. It is very difficult to monitor your speech all the time. Like I say, if she would be fatigued or upset or just generally a case of the flu or something like that, a person with dysarthria, their speech will deteriorate. This is part of the condition.

Q. Is this something that as far as you were able to determine is going to be with her for the rest of her life?

A. I would say there would be some measure of that, yes. There usually is.

Q. Is there any other manifestation of dysarthria?

A. No. Severe dysarthria, a person sounds like they are drunk and a person reacts to them perhaps as an alcoholic or something. It can be very embarrassing.

Q. Will the degree of dysarthria vary with the degree of fatigue or the degree of external stress?

A. Yes.

Q. So, if it were a great deal of stress, her speech would probably be more slurred than if there were less stress?

A. Right. With a person who is dysarthric, they have to continually monitor how they are talking and sounding practically all the time, which in itself is stressful. If you had to think about how you produce every word you would get uptight pretty fast.

As I still had several medical points to discuss with Clark Jameson, the plan was for me to meet him at his office after checking into my hotel. This took longer than I had anticipated, and it was nearly noon before I got to his building. He was waiting for the elevator just as I arrived.

"Dick, good to see you. I called the hotel, but you'd already gone out. Listen, something's come up and I've got to dash off to a meeting. Shouldn't be more than an hour. Meanwhile, I'm leaving you in custody of Claire Glynn, Laura's mother—she's dying to talk to you. Also I thought you might want to see Laura, so I set up an appointment for this afternoon, okay?"

I agreed and went into his office, where Mrs. Glynn was waiting. She was very much as Clark had described her, slender and very attractive, with a look and manner reminiscent of Lena Horne. That she was also a highly intelligent and dynamic woman was just as apparent.

"Mr. Jameson had kindly offered his office as a sitting room. I hope that's all right with you, Doctor."

"Of course, perfectly fine."

Mrs. Glynn took a cigarette case out of her handbag and held it open to me. "No? Well, of course you wouldn't smoke. You know better." She got up to look for an ashtray, her movements graceful and precise. "I must start off by thanking you, Dr. Chodoff. We're very grateful to you for coming out here to testify. That was my main reason for wanting to meet you." She paused. "And also a certain amount of curiosity, I must admit, to see the one surgeon who not only said yes, this was malpractice, but yes, I'll testify to that."

I rearranged myself in one of Clark's leather executive armchairs, feeling somewhat embarrassed under the bright gaze of her large brown eyes.

"What I'm doing is a very normal thing, Mrs. Glynn, just following the dictates of conscience. It seems to me the surgeons who don't might be worthier of your curiosity."

"Well put, Doctor," she said with a rueful smile. "It's fairly obvious, I suppose, that after two years I'm far from reconciled to what happened to Laura."

"It's not an easy thing to accept." I wished, as usual, that I had more than banalities to offer as consolation.

"I keep going over and over it. It's so baffling. This didn't happen in some godforsaken little town. Laura had a good, well-trained surgeon in one of the city's best hospitals. In a more or less civilized country," she went on bitterly, "where you would expect to find at the very least some kind of communication." As she spoke Mrs. Glynn paced the room, every now and then brushing aside a cloud of cigarette smoke. "Do you mind the smoke, Doctor? I know it's bad for me. You're being very restrained not saying so, aren't you?" And again she gave her rather winning melancholy smile.

"Well, yes, actually I am."

She put the cigarette out and sat down on the leather couch opposite me. "It's good of you to—I was going to say talk with me like this, but listen is what I mean."

"Sometimes it's the only thing that helps."

"Don't I know it. One of our problems is that Laura's injury is such a delicate subject—or so people think. Everybody's always skirting round it—I can't even discuss it with my husband. Less with him than anybody, poor Tony. Laura has always been his greatest . . . joy, that's the only word for it. He won't be at the trial tomorrow. He was very much against Laura's husband pressing charges. He just can't bear to be reminded.

"As for me, I can't get it out of my head for a moment. It was all so Kafkaesque, especially the hospital with their iron rules, that unbending insistence on protocol. 'The doctor will have to explain that, Mrs. Glynn.' 'We're not supposed to discuss the medication, Mrs. Glynn.' 'You'll have to ask the head nurse, Mrs. Glynn.' 'It's been noted down, Mrs. Glynn.' 'We'll just have to wait for the doctor, Mrs. Glynn.' It was so obvious something was wrong with Laura from the beginning—a headache that no medication helped, a daze she couldn't seem to rouse herself from. Once we tried walking down the hall with her, Tony and I, and she could hardly make it back to her room, she was so weak. She told the nurses she felt odd—and she certainly sounded it. She kept calling Tony 'Fadder.' And crying when we had to go. Oh, very unlike herself." Mrs. Glynn's face clouded over at the memory. "Can you believe it, there Laura was, in obvious pain, thrashing around in bed, unable to talk straight, and Dr. Ashton saw *nothing* wrong." Mrs. Glynn lit another cigarette and began pacing again.

"I'll never forgive him for not coming back to the hospital when the nurses called him that night. Never. Nor for his dishonesty about it. Tony and I and Marcus, her husband, we all saw that something was wrong with Laura, so did the nurses. Yet afterwards Dr. Ashton kept pretending she'd been all right. And that supercilious manner of his, acting as though he belonged to some exalted species and owed us no explanation. I could not get one straight answer from him. It was like having a conversation with an eel. He was so evasive about what had happened to Laura—it was positively insulting. Oh, I was furious, and I told him so. 'Your evasiveness, your pretenses,' I said, 'are an insult to my intelligence and your profession.' "

Clark Jameson's secretary came in at this point with some papers, and Mrs. Glynn regained her calm.

"You're going out to see Laura?" she asked.

"Yes. I hope it won't disturb her."

"I'm sure it will be fine. They're both anxious to meet you. And Laura's learned to handle situations. Admirably. She's still such a beautiful girl. Yes, even now."

I have spoken to many proud parents in my life, but I don't think I have ever seen anybody light up quite the way Claire Glynn did, talking about her daughter.

"She's tried so hard to pull herself out of this . . . this quagmire. Practicing how to write again all day long, working with a tape recorder to correct her speech. And with such courage, such sweet obstinacy. She doesn't mention it anymore, but her dream, of course, is that she'll be able to pick up her life again. Did Mr. Jameson tell you that Laura had quite an interesting career?"

192

"Yes, a broker's assistant, wasn't she?"

Mrs. Glynn nodded. "She loved it. In fact, she was about to become a full-fledged broker herself. Just before the operation she'd taken the New York Stock Exchange exam. Oh, well—" She broke off, and I knew no words to comfort her.

"One has to be grateful," I finally ventured, "that she did make a certain recovery from the stroke . . ."

Mrs. Glynn gave me a wry look. "Oh, yes, so they all say. Everybody in that hospital was so very quick to assure us that compared to other stroke victims Laura was doing beautifully. But she didn't go into the hospital with a stroke, did she? They seem to forget that interesting little point. And what they don't compare Laura to is Laura. The way she was."

I poured her a glass of water. "This is a difficult question, but how do you compare your daughter with . . . the way she was."

Mrs. Glynn gave a despairing shrug. "Not difficult, Doctor, impossible. We're talking about an exceptionally bright young woman. Now all the brightness, the spontaneity, is gone. Laura has to read something three or four times before she understands it. She knows what she wants to say, but it's hard for her to find the right words. If we talk on the phone at night when she's tired, half the time I can't understand her. Tony used to be in tears listening to her—he couldn't bear it.

"And one can't help worrying about her marriage. Marcus is wonderful with her, but it hasn't been easy for him either. He once told me that he felt guilty because he had encouraged Laura to go to Dr. Miller in the first place. With that noise in her ear she tended to speak in a loud voice, especially on the phone—the sort of thing that can get on a spouse's nerves." She twirled her glass; it was the first abstracted gesture I'd seen.

"Marcus resented Laura's job, a little, I think. Her total absorption in it, I mean. Poor boy, he probably feels guilty about that too. And there Laura is, for the first time a very dependent housewife, and that's a vocation she never had much calling for. Ah, well, it's all a dreadful mess. I don't know how one begins to sort it out." She paused a few moments, lost in thought. "I don't believe she's made her maximum recovery, but it's not easy for her to go on fighting. If they win the case she'll be able to get more therapy—she's become too discouraged lately. She's a gentle soul, like her father. But she's got so much to fight for."

Clark and I did not speak much on the way out to the Carlsons' place. He was preoccupied, worried about the trial, as indeed I was. I hoped I would do a good job as expert witness. Talking with Mrs. Glynn had given another dimension to the case, a different kind of reality. Taken it from the realm of facts to a family.

"Sort of a space age concept, isn't it?" Clark said as we pulled up to the Carlsons' house. "He's quite an architect. I think they used it for weekends until Laura's stroke. Then they moved out here just until she felt she was coping better. Two years later they're still here."

Marcus Carlson came out to greet us, a tall rather professional-looking young man with graying curls and horn-rimmed glasses.

"Glad to meet you, Doctor," he said, shaking my hand. "Hope the traffic wasn't too bad."

We followed him into the house, which as far as I could see was one vast living room—a circular sunken room with a stone fireplace at its center. Laura sat in a chair near the fireplace, composed and waiting. She was indeed a beautiful girl; darker-skinned than her mother, she had the same elegant features, high cheekbones and large almond-shaped eyes. Then as I crossed the room to her I saw the paralysis that held the right side of her face rigid.

"How do you do, Doctor," she said, holding out her left hand to me. "So kind of you to come." She spoke as slowly as Eliza Doolittle practicing the English language. "Do please sit down. You too, Mr. Jameson."

"What can I get you gentlemen to drink?" Marcus Carlson asked.

"Nothing for me, thanks," we both replied, more or less in unison.

"I don't think this should be a long visit. We don't want to tire Laura out," Clark said. "Tomorrow's the big day."

"I shall be fine tomorrow," Laura said in that careful distinct voice, but I saw the uncertain glance she gave her husband, and the way he quickly went to sit down beside her.

"It's a great house. Your design, I understand, Mr. Carlson?" I said, and we chatted for a few moments about contemporary architecture.

"Dick, if there's anything specific you want to discuss with Laura . . ." Clark was giving me my cue, and reluctantly, as gently as I knew how, I asked what she remembered of the first operation.

"Well," she said, "very little except the pain in my head. Marcus was there, and my parents. And I remember being upset because the whistling was still in my ear." She stopped a moment and then continued slowly. "Dr. Ashton came in and he said that I was probably depressed because I *thought* I could still hear the noise."

"The next day her headache was much worse," her husband said.

Laura nodded, frowning a little. "It wasn't just an ordinary headache. It was the whole side of my head. I stayed in bed because the . . . pills didn't help. The pain was ex—" She paused, searching for the word.

"Excruciating," Marcus supplied.

"Yes—that's right," Laura said but made no attempt to repeat the word. "My aunt was planning to visit me, and I called Marcus at his office to tell him not to bring her along, that I felt too bad. And that's when I discovered I couldn't talk. That is, I was talking, but the words were all wrong. It was . . . gibberish."

"I went right out to the hospital as soon as I heard her," Marcus told me.

"It was very strange," Laura said. "Like a dream, a fog. They, my mother and father and Marcus, were on the other side. I was aware that they were trying to rouse me, and the nurse was shouting, but I could hardly hear them and my eyes kept closing." Laura's words were coming faster and beginning to slur.

"Slow down, darling," her husband said anxiously.

She nodded and took a deep breath. "The last thing I recall was that I was strapped to the bed. I didn't realize it then. I only knew that I was very uncomfortable, but I couldn't move around freely . . ."

"After the second operation?" Clark said.

Laura shook her head. "I don't remember much. I'm told I was in the intensive-care unit for some time. Later I remember that every night I would buzz for the nurse and she would come in but I couldn't talk. So she would ask me questions and finally she would get around to saying, "Do you have a headache?" and I would nod yes and she would get a pill and I would take it."

"You still couldn't speak at that point?" I asked.

"No. . . . I was in the . . ." She looked at her husband for help.

"Stroke center," Marcus replied.

"Yes—I was there for two weeks, and when I left, there was only one thing I could say." She paused, with a wry look that reminded me of her mother. " 'Sip the milk.' "

"What about your right leg?" I asked. "You were walking when you were discharged from the hospital?"

Laura hesitated. Her expression, which until now had been one of total concentration, gave way to a brief bitterness. "When I walked I would go into the wall, the right wall. I couldn't keep to a straight line. Now . . . it is still weak. I can't dance anymore, but at least I am not walking into the wall." Laura turned round to pet the dog that had jumped up to sit beside her, and it was dismaying to suddenly see the right side of her face again. She had been sitting in an attitude that I imagine she'd cultivated since the stroke, keeping her good profile to the company. "Before, I could not feel my dog's hair at all. Now I can a little." She went on to say something else I did not quite catch.

"Slow down," Marcus told her. "It's hard—Laura forgets and tries to speak too quickly."

"I said," Laura spoke very slowly, a look of frustration and embarrassment on her face, "it is like wearing a glove—the feeling of my hand. The same with my face." She touched, as though shielding it, her right cheek. "It is numb, that whole side. I cannot wink my eye, for instance."

"Well—a good thing, I'd say," Clark said, with what for him was a rather heavy humor.

"Have you considered more therapy for your hand?" I asked.

"The physical therapist at the hospital said the best thing would be doing dishes—the hot water." Laura glanced at Marcus, and fleetingly I recognized her mother's rueful little smile. She then asked if we wouldn't like something to drink. At least I gathered this is what she said, from Clark's reply, for her speech was becoming difficult to understand. Clearly she was tired. There were long pauses—as though each word had separately to be found, brought back from some faraway recess of her mind, and not every attempt was successful.

Marcus, at Clark's suggestion, took us on a tour of the house, and we left shortly afterward. Back in town, Clark and I had dinner, but I remember nothing about the evening. From the time we left the young couple and through a restless night, I experienced a great discomfort in my soul. I had, I don't quite know how to describe it, say, a universal ache.

I kept thinking of the ancient medical proverb, the most basic of our ethics: *Primum non nocere*—First, do no harm. It seemed to me that Laura Carlson had been done not only great harm, but a grave injustice. To have been offered no decent compensation, to have to appear in court to prove an obvious injury—this surely was to turn her experience into a nightmare of classic proportions. Why can't the medical profession find a more humane way to treat those we've injured? So went my thoughts until the next morning when the trial began.

Clark Jameson's direct examination of Laura worked well, and the jury appeared to be a sympathetic one. His low-keyed approach, devoid of the histrionics used by some plaintiffs' attorneys, was in perfect accord with Laura's slow and unemotional recital of the events that followed her operation.

Then came the defense attorney, a bright young man who, by some very fancy maneuvering, tried to plant doubts in the minds of the jury without seeming to attack Laura. As he did not want to risk antagonizing the jury by an outright challenge of her story, he conducted his examination with the greatest tact. Innuendo took the place of blanket statements; subtly he questioned the accuracy of her memory, sympathetically he suggested that her postoperative headache and somnolence were a reaction to the anesthesia. With exaggerated politesse and discretion he went on to imply that her neurological symptoms were the result of a disturbed psyche, caused by strange surroundings and highly exaggerated apprehension.

Though Laura began to have trouble finding words and her speech slurred under the pressure, she maintained her composure and continued with a halting but unconfused account of her bewildering postoperative hours. It was a most poignant and dramatic testimony, and clearly I was not the only one to think so, for there was a kind of charged silence in the courtroom. The judge, a portly and distinguished white-haired gentleman, was leaning slightly forward to listen to Laura, and it was apparent that most of the jurors were sympathetic. So much so, in fact, that when she described her inability to speak and move her right side, the defense attorney quickly stopped his examination and dismissed her from the witness box.

Dr. Ashton was the same artful dodger in his courtroom testimony as in his deposition. He glossed over his negligence, emphasized the irrelevancies of the case and minimized the injuries. He blamed "inadvertently" tying off the internal carotid artery on its size; his failure to recognize Laura's stroke, on its slow appearance. Aided and abetted by his mendacious expert witnesses, Dr. Ashton insisted the patient had "been without complaints" for thirty hours after the first operation. He complimented himself on restoring flow into the internal carotid system in Laura's second surgical procedure, "done with some difficulty but successfully," and stated that following this she was "quite alert."

Accustomed as I had grown to appearing in court, I felt quite anxious that morning. It seemed an unusually long time before I was finally called to the witness stand. I swore to tell the truth, the whole truth and nothing but the truth, so help me God. Then, under Clark's direct examination, I gave the jury my unreserved opinions of the defendant doctor's inordinate negligence. I testified that I considered Dr. Ashton's initial decision to operate on Laura Carlson morally questionable; that her subsequent stroke was due to the ligation of her internal carotid artery, a mistake that could not be condoned since no vessel in the neck, regardless of size or position, should be tied off without positive identification. In conclusion, I stated that the doctor's disregard of his patient's neurological symptoms and his failure to return to the hospital at 10 P.M. when the nurses called him were totally unethical. Had he reoperated at that time, the plaintiff would have suffered far less brain damage, perhaps none at all.

The defense attorney in his cross-examination of me let go the usual barrage of slanderous questions, more than usual, since he was well aware that he needed to distract the jury from his indefensible case. I was asked if I got paid on a contingency-fee basis, whether I advertised my services in legal journals and how I had become involved in the case. Then he overplayed his hand.

"Doctor, you live in Philadelphia, several thousand miles from here. How does it come about that you're in Kansas testifying in this case?"

There was an immediate objection to this question by Clark Jameson, and a discussion at the bench. The judge dismissed the jury at this point so that the discussion could continue without prejudicing them.

"You opened the area with your question," he told the defense attorney. "You've got to let him answer any way he wants to." Then he turned to me and said, "Doctor, if the jury were present how would you answer that question?"

I thought for a minute or two. "Your Honor, I think every injured plaintiff has as much right to an expert witness as the defendant doctor. So, Your Honor, I guess I would have to say that it's a shame there wasn't a surgeon closer to Kansas than Philadelphia who was willing to testify on behalf of a young woman who has been so grievously injured by surgical negligence."

"When the jury returns," the judge said, "tell them exactly what you've just told me."

The jury was recalled, and I answered the question as I had been instructed by the judge. The few subsequent questions asked me by the defense attorney were inconsequential, and I was soon finished and excused.

The next day, shortly after I got back to Philadelphia, Clark Jameson called to say that the jury had brought in a verdict for Laura. "And I've a message for you from Claire Glynn."

"Oh?"

"She said to tell you thank heavens for Richard Chodoff and Edmund Burke."

I confess I was as puzzled as I was pleased. It was Paula who finally figured out Mrs. Glynn's allusion to that eighteenth-century English statesman:

"There is but one law for all, namely the law which governs all law, the law of our Creator, the law of humanity, justice . . ."

11

ON OUR TWELFTH wedding anniversary, the Habers surprised Paula and me with a party on a hired schooner. It was a splendid evening, which turned into a surprise for everybody when Dan discovered that the crew had been celebrating, too, and were in no shape to navigate us back into the harbor. As a result we sailed in misty circles until dawn, moving slowly through a kind of Outward Bound atmosphere that was as lovely as it was strange.

Michael Waring was one of the friends along on this anniversary excursion, and during a lull in the festivities, when I was chatting with Dan and Beatrice, I saw Paula in earnest conversation with him.

"They're talking business, I bet you anything," Beatrice said. "Hey, don't you people ever stop to party?"

"Paula, for shame," Dan said with mock opprobrium. "A face and a dress that befit a princess, and this is how you celebrate your anniversary—discussing malpractice?"

"My fault," Michael said. "I'm the one who started it."

"No, he didn't," Paula said, smiling at me. "Anyway, shop talk belongs in the celebration, doesn't it, Dick? If it weren't for Michael we'd never have met, let alone be an old married couple."

"Only half of us fits that description," I said, thinking how remarkably young and beautiful she looked, sitting there in the hazy moonlight. "And I promise you, even if Michael hadn't sent you to see me, we'd be together today anyway. It's kismet."

Beatrice heaved a big theatrical sigh. "Tell me, what's it like being married twelve years to such a Lothario?"

"You don't have to answer that question before consulting with your attorney," Michael said, and everybody laughed.

Though Paula joined in this light bantering, I caught the grave, reflective expression in her eyes, and after the Habers went aft, where somebody was playing a guitar, I sat down with her and Michael. It was easy enough to guess what case they'd been discussing.

"Anything new on Lois Schiller?" I asked, naming a client of Michael's I'd agreed to testify for, a young woman dying of cancer.

"Michael's going out to San Francisco for the pretrial examination," Paula said. "She's back in the hospital again."

"For the final time, I'm afraid," Michael said.

Paula gave a little shiver, and I took off my jacket and wrapped it around her. "That better?"

She nodded. "Sorry. For some reason this case has really got to me. Here we are, we have each other, our life together, and there's that poor girl. It's so damn unfair, she never even had a chance. Sometimes I think this is the worst case yet."

"In many ways it is," Michael said.

"When are you going out to California?" I asked him.

"Early next week. It seems fairly certain she won't live long enough to make it to court, so I'm going to do a videotape of her deposition. It's the only way she'll testify at her trial."

The Schiller case was, as Paula said, one of the worst. In my opinion the plaintiff was treated with unparalleled nonchalance. Yet not only did the defendant doctor deny any charge of negligence, he had as his expert witness a prominent professor of surgery, ready and willing to fly in the face of all incontrovertible medical facts in order to protect his colleague.

Lois Schiller, wife of a Navy man and young mother of two children, discovered lumps in her breast and went to see her family doctor in the clinic of a naval hospital. This general practitioner, because of a naval regulation, was not permitted to order mammograms, but he felt she should have one and he arranged a surgical consultation for her in the same hospital. The surgeon, however, made no attempt to investigate Mrs. Schiller's breast lumps for a possible diagnosis of cancer. He neither aspirated for cytologic study nor did a biopsy, nor did he order a mammogram. He merely examined her breasts, told her the lumps were fibrocystic, not to worry, and to come back in six months. Because of increasing pain and discomfort, Mrs. Schiller returned in four months. Once again the surgeon reassured her without recommending any diagnostic procedures. Three more months passed, and the patient who by now was experiencing a great deal of pain, returned to the doctor to ask him to do something. He said he did not think it necessary but he would send her for a mammogram if it would make her feel any better. Mammography was finally done, and Mrs. Schiller was diagnosed as having advanced carcinoma of the breast with involvement of the axillary nodes. Within a very short time, despite both mastectomy and chemotherapy, the disease metastasized.

When Michael got back from San Francisco, he stopped by my office to tell me that he had succeeded in filming Mrs. Schiller's deposition.

"She managed to get through all the questioning?" I asked.

"Beautifully, though God knows how. She's weak as a kitten and full of medication."

"How much longer do they give her?"

"A month, maybe two. The cancer's everywhere now." Michael sighed, and busied himself searching for one of his small thin cigars and then for his lighter. "What can I tell you? It was a very grim scene. She's just bones and huge blue eyes, wearing a bandana with yellow daisies so nobody will know she's completely bald. For all she's been through, she's still like a young girl—soft-spoken, so overwhelmed by everything."

"Any family there?"

"Her mother was taking care of the kids, but Schiller was there. He's just like Lois, a nice mild fellow in a daze, he doesn't seem to have quite absorbed what's happened."

"She knows you're going to request permission to play the videotape in court?"

"Oh, sure. In fact, I think it's something she's counting very much on." Michael paused. "It's interesting, you know. Lois never really verbalized her feelings. Her main emotion was this . . . bafflement at what was happening, so I was surprised at how determined she was to get the filming done. She was so distrait and weak, and yet she held herself together for it. She felt she was needlessly dying and she wanted it made public."

Six weeks later Lois Schiller died. In December, five months after her death, I went out to San Francisco to testify at the trial. As the defendant doctor was a government employee, the case was tried in a federal court and was, in accord with the Federal Court Tort Claims Act, trial without jury.

I do not think I am likely ever to forget the atmosphere of that trial. The court with its dark wood paneling and empty jury box was so impressive and so quiet it seemed like a stage set. As for the characters, they were a dignified, conservative-looking judge; Dr. Bellows, the defendant, with an impervious expression and a stubborn set to his mouth; Dr. Jefferson, the defendant's expert witness, who looked like the busy, prominent surgeon he is; and Dr. Simpson, the earnest young general practitioner who'd first seen Lois Schiller and who, like me, was a witness for the plaintiff. Accustomed as I was to a more modest municipal court and to an attentive row of jurors, I was very conscious of the empty jury box as I listened to testimony that mocked truth and honor and gave that imposing court a hollow grandeur.

To meet the normal standards of care there were such well-known basic steps Dr. Bellows should have taken when diagnosing Mrs. Schiller's breast lumps that the charge of negligence seemed inarguable to me. Yet the defendant and his expert witness shamelessly quibbled with the questions put to them.

Dr. Bellows insisted that he found no indications to obtain any objective data to confirm or rule out his diagnosis of a fibrocystic disease. When he was asked if he ought not to have had Mrs. Schiller return after her menses in order to reexamine her breasts, he said he told her that if she found any change, if things didn't get better, to let him know and he would promptly check her, approximately one week after a period. Yet what came out under further cross-examination by Michael Waring was:

Q. Doctor, you wrote down recheck in six months. You did not write down recheck in one week or two weeks. You didn't write down any of that, did you?

A. No, I told her to recheck in six months unless things don't get better.

Q. It is your testimony to this Court that you have a specific recollection of having told her to come back in a week or two if things hadn't changed, even though you recorded on your consultation right here recheck in six months?

A. My specific recollection concerns all breast patients. I tell all my breast patients exactly the same thing, depending on their individual findings.

The surgeon maintained that when Mrs. Schiller did return for a second visit he found her condition "even better," and that now "there was no lump." When Michael reminded him of Mrs. Schiller's continued pain and complaint of a lump in her breast and another under her arm, Dr. Bellows' reply was, "She had the lump under the arm. As far as the lump in the breast is concerned, it is a matter of what term you choose to use. I still maintain that on the basis of my examination there was not a lump present. Just because a patient says a lump is there that does not mean a physician is going to find one. The physician, fortunately in most cases, knows more than the patient does and is better able to assess objective findings than the patient."

Even when confronted with the hardly moot question of a longer life for Mrs. Schiller had there been an immediate diagnosis and operation, the defendant, impassive as ever, continued his meaningless hedging: "It is possible she would have lived later than that date, yes; however, using statistics and size and type of tumor is very treacherous, because all of the numbers you are talking about, probabilities and possibilities, are retrospective."

Perhaps more shocking still were some of the statements made by

Dr. Jefferson, the eminent breast specialist who testified on the defendant's behalf. He stoutly announced that he "would have done just what was done." When asked if he was aware that Dr. Simpson had not been permitted to order a mammogram and so had sent Mrs. Schiller to Dr. Bellows specifically for evaluation of the breast lumps, the witness replied, "I don't know what the doctor was doing. It seems to me he was asking for a further opinion in an area where he is not sure of it. It would seem to me that if he wanted to get a mammogram, he could have ordered one before he ever sent her to Dr. Bellows, but I don't know what transpired in the Navy medical realm."

One of the most interesting moments to me was when Dr. Jefferson, an acknowledged authority on breast cancer, was asked whether he agreed with his own published statement "A palpable mass should either be aspirated for cytologic study or excised for histologic study, regardless of whether it appears to be on xeroradiography or mammography." Blandly the doctor replied, "Yes, I think we all agree with what the book says." And yet he persisted, under oath, in protecting his colleague:

Q. Would you state whether or not you have an opinion as to the standard of care exercised by Dr. Bellows on both those occasions?

A. I think the standard of care exercised by him was perfectly adequate.

When Michael called me to the stand he asked for the approximate number of breast operations I had performed over my career. I explained that as I had been practicing surgery for forty-two years, the total was around four hundred, and well over a thousand for benign breast lesions. Asked for the date of the last breast surgery, I replied, "I have a patient in the hospital now on whom I did a modified radical mastectomy last Tuesday."

Q. Doctor, when was the last time you did a surgical biopsy for breast cancer?

A. Well, this was the last biopsy for cancer. This was

followed by a mastectomy. The last patient I had who had a breast problem before this was about twelve days ago and I did a bilateral biopsy which turned out to be bilateral cysticmastitis.

I was then requested to "clearly document" what in my opinion were Dr. Bellows' breaches of the standard of care Mrs. Schiller should have received.

A. No attempt was made in any way to make a diagnosis. There was a diagnosis of fibrocystic disease which, I guess, was by osmosis. In my opinion, in a mass like this, an attempt should be made to aspirate it. If the typical fluid is obtained which you usually see in patients with cysticmastitis, sort of a cloudy greenish, dirty-looking fluid, and that mass disappears and does not come back, I would decide to examine the patient a month or two later. Then I think I could be absolutely satisfied that this patient has a benign cyst and nothing further need be done except for an occasional periodic observation, which I do and which I think should be done in patients like this every six months.

Given the fact that the needle was put in, and no fluid obtained, immediately then a mammogram should have been ordered to see whether the suspicion of malignancy which had been aroused by the patient's history, by your examination, and by the fact that aspiration did not yield any fluid, then a mammogram would help you in making the diagnosis. It will either say, yes, this shows evidence of malignancy or not. Even if the mammogram is not specific and even if the mammogram does not say that this looks like cancer, it is incumbent on every surgeon to remove the thing and have it under the microscope so you know what it is. There is no way of guessing what lumps in the breast are. There are too many things that can fool you and I myself have seen too many patients with typical cysticmastitis where the cancer runs deeply. You cannot guess with that. You are playing with a patient's life. Once you take a biopsy and get that tissue out, there is no more guessing. It is an area of cystic disease, primarily fibrotic, and you are finished, and if it is cancer, you go ahead and take it out; so, I think that pretty well covers it.

Q. Now, I am going to ask you if you have an opinion, based upon reasonable medical probability, as to the effect, if any, of the early diagnosis of cancer in Mrs. Schiller's left breast and treatment between November of '78 and March of 1979? Do you have an opinion?

A. Yes.

Q. What is your opinion in respect to the delay?

A. I think the delay denied her any chance of survival. I think it shortened her life tremendously and was directly responsible for her death.

One of the most honest and touching testimonies I ever heard from a doctor was given by the plaintiff's other witness, Dr. Simpson. This young general practitioner had left the naval hospital to go into private practice and was still obviously disturbed by the regulation which had kept him from ordering Mrs. Schiller's mammogram. Indeed, as his self-accusatory statements showed, he was deeply troubled by his own role in the case.

THE COURT. Would it be presumptuous of you, as a medical doctor, to suggest on referring the matter to a surgeon for evaluation the possibility of mammography?

THE WITNESS. Well . . . I certainly am not blameless in this instance. I have spent many sleepless nights wondering about my own part in this whole thing. I should have, let's put it that way. I saw that lady numerous times after I referred her to Dr. Bellows. I passed off that problem as his problem and failed to deal with it. Had I felt the mass subsequently, had I been continuously concerned about it, I certainly could have called him up on the telephone and urged him to get a mammography on her. Those are things that I could have done that I did not do. It seems to be common feeling that was Dr. Bellows' province and that, for whatever reason, I, perhaps am legally blameless, but still I think that . . . there undoubtedly was an obligation on my part to do things that I did not do and, if nothing else, to suggest to Mrs. Schiller that perhaps the care she was receiving in the Navy was not what I considered adequate and suggest discreetly that she go someplace else and get a second opinion, you know, numerous things that could have been done that were not done for that whole eight months between the time I first examined her and the tumor was discovered; so, in answer to your question, I probably should have done just exactly that and did not.

The judge's reply to Dr. Simpson was, I suppose, a pretty clear indication of how the court was thinking.

THE COURT. Well, you may be a little hard on yourself, Doctor. In your own defense, I think it proper to observe in the four subsequent visits that she had, she had other complaints, but apparently none of them related to her breast.

To the young doctor's enormous credit he refused this invitation to be whitewashed, and though it was not he who was on trial he continued to confess the guilt he felt.

THE WITNESS. But the consultation was still in the file and it is generally considered good form to review patients' records and kind of keep track of all the problems going on. I either didn't do that, being too busy, or whatever, or I did it and chose to ignore it. I can't right now tell you this. I was at the time powerless, I think, to do anything about it. I still couldn't order a mammogram and I think that is my justification. . . .

But Dr. Simpson's display of self-incriminating integrity apparently did not impress the court. Nor did the videotape that showed a skeletal Lois Schiller propped up in her hospital bed, wearing a bright bandana and making so valiant an effort with her testimony. Had there been a jury to see this final, poignant proof of negligence, I am certain the verdict could not have been otherwise than for the plaintiff. The court, however, ruled in favor of the defendant doctor.

In the hope that Lois Schiller's words might after all reach a jury, the following has been excerpted from her filmed deposition.

LOIS MARGARET SCHILLER, called for examination, having first been duly sworn according to law, was examined and testified as follows:

COUNSEL FOR THE PLAINTIFF. First of all, let the record show that this deposition is being made at Mrs. Schiller's bedside at the United States Naval Hospital in San Francisco, California. Mrs. Schiller, if you will state your full name, I would ask that you look towards the camera. Now would you state your full name.

A. Lois Margaret Schiller.

Q. I believe your husband is also here in the room. How long have you been married?

A. Ten years in July.

Q. I'm going to try to avoid asking you separate questions because I'm trying to avoid prolonging this deposition. So would you tell us the background of the circumstances which led to the filing of your claim which is now pending?

A. It all started in November of 1968 when I found lumps—

Q. November of '68, Mrs. Schiller, or '78?

A. I'm sorry, '78, excuse me. I went to see my family doctor after finding lumps in my breast.

Q. Let me ask you this for the purpose of the record, too, Mrs. Schiller, are you under any medication tonight?

A. I haven't taken much at all because I can't keep it down. I had some earlier this afternoon, but they say it will wear off in three hours.

Q. You had some tests today, did you?

A. Yes, I had a brain scan today.

Q. Brain scan? This deposition, for the record, started at 7:22 P.M. and it is now 7:30. So we're about eight minutes into your testimony, and I will ask you, if I ask you a question and you don't understand it or you don't remember, don't be, you know, ashamed to say so.

A. Right, okay.

Q. Now, the first time the discussion of a lump on your breast was held with Dr. Simpson was when?

A. This was November of 1978. I went in there to get it examined. I had one under my arm and one in my left breast. He found the other two that were in the right breast.

Q. All right. What, if anything, did he recommend?

A. He made an appointment for the surgeon downstairs to see me. That was Thomas Bellows.

Q. What if anything occurred there—what did he say, what did you say to him?

A. He said it was—he examined me thoroughly, said it was nothing to worry about, it was fibrocystic is what he called it. He gave me Vitamin A pills and said to come back in six months if it was still bothering me.

Q. Now, by bothering you I take it you are referring to your breast and under your arm?

A. Right. He said there wasn't a whole lot they could do about fibrocystic.

Q. What, if anything, did you say to him when he gave you this advice?

A. Well, I thought he knew what he was talking about, I thought he was right. But then, of course, later on when it kept getting sore—I came back in three months because it was bothering me.

Q. How was it bothering you?

A. It was hard to sleep at night because I couldn't sleep on my side.

Q. Did you have any pain?

A. Yes, very definite pain with it. I told him again, Dr. Bellows, that I, it was very painful.

Q. Refer to the part of your body involved.

A. Okay. The two lumps that I went in to see about to

begin with were the ones that were painful, one under my arm and one under my left breast. The other two apparently had disappeared. So, anyway, he told me again there was very little he could do.

Q. Did he recommend surgery?

A. Oh, no, nothing. He again said it was fibrocystic and just to come back and see him.

Q. Did he recommend a biopsy?

A. No, he did not.

Q. Did he recommend a mammogram?

A. No, that was not recommended, either. When I went back—well, I told him also that both my grandparents had died of cancer.

Q. You told Dr. Bellows that?

A. Right, but this didn't seem to make any difference. He didn't, doesn't seem to be anything he could do about it. So then when I went back the third time—

Q. Which was when?

A. This is June, 1979.

Q. What was your condition when you went back as compared to what your condition was in March?

A. It was much worse. The breast was swollen and it was hard inside, it was a big hard knot . . . and I was very concerned about it. Plus the fact that I just learned that my grandmother had died of breast cancer. I knew she had died of cancer. I didn't know at that time it was breast cancer. So I was upset when I saw Dr. Bellows, not upset, but I told him I was tired of messing around, I wanted a mammogram, that I wanted something done. And he said, well, he didn't think there was anything, you know—

Q. Did he think you needed it?

A. He said, I don't think you need it, but if it makes you feel better I'll send you over and have a mammogram done. And then he made an appointment. So I went over. It was within an hour after I got back that he called me. He said there was a possibility of cancer in the left breast and that he wanted to see me the next day. I went over there. He had the admission papers all written out and everything. At this time he examined me again, saying that this lump that I had then—

Q. Meaning under your arm?

A. Okay, the one that I had all the time was a new one. I didn't think he was right, because I knew it was the same lump . . .

Q. Did Dr. Bellows following the surgery have any discussion with you relative to the earlier visit you made to him at which time he described your condition as being fibrocystic?

A. No. In fact, there was no comment at all from Dr. Bellows. No apology for any misdiagnosing, nothing. In fact, the night before my surgery he even said, it's still a fifty-fifty chance of taking off the breast, and the surgical nurse came in and . . . she says Dr. Bellows did tell you that there was a ninety percent chance of taking off the breast.

Q. Mrs. Schiller, I have to ask you some questions now which in view of the fact that you are in the hospital and . . . getting I.V. fluid, and . . . I know this is the last thing in the world you want done is to have your testimony taken right now, it may seem silly to ask you how you feel, but I must go back following the surgery when your breast was removed, how did you physically and emotionally feel following the operation?

A. Well, it was a big loss certainly, but I was under the impression that they had gotten all the cancer . . . so I was, you know . . .

Q. Relieved?

A. Relieved, right . . . . But . . . losing a breast is a big adjustment . . . . It took a while to adjust to it, but I . . . got over it. Excuse me, I have to get some water.

Q. You want me to stop for a few minutes, Mrs. Schiller? Would you like a break for a few minutes?

A. Yes.

(Whereupon a short recess was taken).

Q. Mrs. Schiller, from the time following the breast surgery what has been your state of health? Trace very quickly if you will what your health has been and leading up to your very confinement here tonight.

A. Well, of course they put me on chemotherapy, which tends to put your health downhill, too, because it nauseates you a lot. I was on chemotherapy for ten months. Then I entered the hospital in May . . . . I was in here for three weeks trying to get the calcium down. It was nausea, I was sick. Then I was out—I was in quite good health. In September I had radiation, which put me under quite—

Q. Let me stop you for a moment. I know you have this scarf on your head, what has happened to your hair?

A. . . . well, I have none.

Q. Can you take it off so they can photograph that?

A. This is due to chemotherapy and radiation both.

Q. You can put that back on now if you will. How long has it been that you lost your hair?

A. Well, the first chemotherapy it got thin. Then with the second bout of chemotherapy . . . it just went in about a month's time. It was strong chemotherapy.

Q. From the period when those chemotherapy treatments stopped until . . . you came back here to the naval hospital, how did you feel during that period of time?

A. Other than being sick from the chemotherapy I was under the impression, you know, everything was going fine

Q. I understand.

A. That's when it hit the liver . . . that's when I was hospitalized.

Q. You say your cancer has spread, how do you know?

A. This is from bone scans.

Q. Did they tell you that?

A. Yes.

Q. Where have you been told that the cancer has spread?

A. Okay, it's in my ribs, in here, it's under my arm here. . . . And it's in my head and also in my pelvis.

Q. By "head" you mean brain?

A. No, not in the brain, bone.

Q. . . . I see, skull?

213

A. In the skull.

Q. No further questions.

Attorney for the Plaintiff. I haven't anything further. Thank you very much.

The Witness. I'm glad that you could come.

12

SHORTLY AFTER THE Schiller case, Paula graduated law school and
subsequently passed her bar exam with flying colors. As soon as we
heard this good news I took her on a well-deserved holiday. We left
the apartment just the way it was, stacks of books and papers
everywhere, and ran off on a ten-day Caribbean cruise. It was a fine
celebration, because now, with a law degree as well as her medical
background, Paula was, as she said, "a true hybrid, at any rate a
potentially more helpful one." Such is the chiaroscuro quality of
life that one moves constantly from shadow to sunshine.

As I pause now to reflect on my thirteen-year journey from the
operating room to the witness stand, I am aware that today there is a
somewhat different, healthier atmosphere. In part this is due, I
believe, to the way the press has, over the past several years, focused
more directly on the medical-malpractice problems.

Some of my colleagues were taken aback by an article that quoted
the testimony of hospital authorities in a hearing before the New
York State Assembly. These officials stated that in approximately ten
percent of the malpractice cases coming to suits, the medical
records had been altered. They admitted that hospitals routinely
allowed doctors who were being sued to go over their charts. Unlike
my friend Dan, I was not surprised by these statistics, for I had been
involved in cases where handwriting experts proved that portions of
a medical file had been changed. Indeed, I remember that in one

such case the plaintiff's attorney discovered that the defendant doctor had taken the chart home for a week after he learned that he was being sued for malpractice.

Publicity was also given to an extensive investigation into the quality of surgery. Sponsored by the American College of Surgeons and the American Surgical Association, this study revealed that forty-seven percent of the 1,696 surgical deaths or complications investigated were preventable. Adding their statistics to this new drive for public enlightenment, the Department of Health, Education and Welfare published the result of their investigations: one third of the estimated twenty million surgical procedures performed, they stated, are unnecessary. The AMA replied in headlines, claiming that this figure was "grossly exaggerated"; that there was only a "tiny amount" of unnecessary surgery. The press also reported on a three-year study done by Blue Cross and Blue Shield of Greater New York which showed that thirty percent of the surgical cases had not had second opinions to confirm the need for operation. Tonsillectomies and orthopedic, gynecological and urological procedures were cited as the most common examples of unnecessary surgery.

The newspapers also, for the first time, gave complete coverage to a malpractice trial in which there had been the sort of dishonorable backstage maneuverings I had so often encountered. Apparently, suit was filed against a prominent orthopedic surgeon by a patient who after a delicate back operation found he had lost bowel and bladder control and been rendered sexually impotent. Once the trial was under way the defendant doctor tried to scare off the expert witnesses scheduled to testify against him. Employing the tactics of a mobster, he used a network of doctor friends to "deliver the message."

One physician was informed by his "mentor" that he should "tread lightly" and "this is not a threat but . . ." The nonthreat was that his testimony was "going to be transcribed and disseminated to his local medical society and to the American Academy of Orthopedic Surgeons."

The other witness, a young neurosurgeon, received the word from his professor, the former chief of neurosurgery at a large teaching hospital. The message was that "it might not be particularly good for the doctor to testify in an out-of-state medical malpractice trial with an impending appearance before the American Board of Neurological Surgery for the oral portion of his certification examinations." Though the young doctor feared he might be blackballed by the Board for being a "violator of the conspiracy of silence," he did not change his plan to testify, because he felt his "evaluation of the case was correct." "I don't want to take on the whole medical community," he said, "I don't want to take anybody on. I just thought what was done was wrong."

The case, which resulted in the court reversing the jury's verdict for the defendant doctor and ordering a new trial, stirred up medical communities everywhere. I remember it was one of the few times I saw Dan's rather detached concern turn into anger.

"Who the hell does he think he is, Al Capone?" he said, referring to the defendant doctor. "First he butchers some poor guy and then he *threatens* the witnesses."

"It's only another version of the story I've been telling you for years now," I pointed out.

"Yes, well—" Dan tugged at his mustache fitfully—"this is different somehow. The concern with whitewashing a Fellow is wrong, but doctors think they're being good, at least to each other. This is like you getting the shaft from Jefferson, this is bribery, blackmail, inner-gang bullying—I don't know what-all, except it's really rotten."

Clearly, the widespread publicity of the malpractice crisis has inspired a certain amount of change in the medical attitude. None of us, after all, wants to see the entire profession discredited by so small a minority of inept men. Doctors have begun writing articles urging patients not to be too intimidated to ask for the information they need. Hospitals are printing leaflets for the patient, clearly stating his rights. Patients are being advised to do what basic investigation they can: to make sure a doctor is Board-certified in his specialty; to inquire about his hospital privileges; to explore alternative therapies; and, when in doubt, to ask for a second opinion. In some communities physicians and patients are getting together to hold round-table discussions in an attempt to solve the communication problem that exists between them.

But the most meaningful change of all is that now there are more doctors who feel a greater responsibility to speak out on behalf of the injured patient. A resident in a metropolitan hospital recently announced that he and his fellow residents would give evidence to document what he called a deliberate pattern of neglect and murderously low levels of medical support. The doctors had already formed a review committee and planned to encourage victims of malpractice and their families to seek redress in the courts. "We'll give these people the information that they need to build a case on," the young doctor said, "even if it means implicating ourselves."

These changes, though slight, are nonetheless signs which are heartening to Paula and me. And Dan. For, several weeks after the "Al Capone" affair, Dan called me at home one night.

"I want to talk to you, Dick," he said, sounding oddly agitated.

"Nothing wrong, I hope."

"No. Yes. Listen, I'd really like to see you now, tonight. Is that okay? Are you and Paula busy?"

"No, it's fine. Come right over." Such terse dialogue was not at all Dan's style, and I was perplexed and worried. I couldn't imagine what had happened since I'd last seen him.

"I've got something to show you," he said by way of greeting. "I still can't believe it's real except here it is in black print." He was waving, like some rabid politician, a copy of a magazine called *The American Lawyer*.

"Have you seen this? It's an old issue. I want you to read it. It's an interview of this defense lawyer, written by Connie Bruck. No, wait, I'm going to read it to you."

"Calm down, will you?" I said, almost laughing. I couldn't remember ever, not even in our student days, seeing Dan in such a state, his wiry hair standing out all over his head. "Go on, sit down. I'll get you a drink. And what are you doing with *The American Lawyer*?"

He gave me a brief grin. "Stole it from Michael. You know his father's coming in for surgery? Well, Michael wanted to talk, so I

218

stopped in at his office and while I was waiting I picked up this—this thing," he said, waving the magazine again. "You sit down, Dick, go on, sit." And, loosening his tie, Dan gave me an agitated orator's reading from an article about defense attorney John Bower:

"Bower and Gardner is probably the largest and many say the best defense firm specializing in torts in the New York area. Most of Bower's clients are insurance companies, self-insured hospitals and drug companies. Bower prizes his firm's reputation as being made up of 'hard-nosed, tough, litigious people,' who are cast in his own mold. 'Settlements are fertile,' he says. 'They beget other settlements. If we are known as bastards who never settle, then plaintiffs' lawyers will look to sue others." Bower buttresses this pragmatism with his personal philosophy about malpractice: 'Professional men have the right to be wrong.'

"Now hear this," Dan said.

"Probably no group of individuals rouses Bower's ire more than plaintiffs' expert witnesses in medical malpractice cases. Most of them, he asserts, are 'whores.' He puts them in a different category from most experts for the defense—who, he insists, are honorable—and argues that they are much better paid.

"For the past 20 years, Bower has been exhorting the insurance industry to set up a computerized clearing-house to keep records of all these experts' testimony. But to no avail. 'The insurance industry couldn't fart together after a lunch of beans,' Bower complains. So he has kept such a bank in his own firm, collecting dossiers on plaintiffs' 'regulars.' Like many lawyers on both sides of the bar, John Bower takes pleasure in characterizing himself as a hired gun, an arch-combatant sent out to do battle in the 'last remaining arena of the gladiators.' The wartime hero he once was, in fact, seems very much in evidence in his legal practice. He adapts easily to the roles in this game (the plaintiff is the enemy), delights in its strategies and manipulations, an even uses wartime language: 'Don't peripherally waste your bullets,' he says. 'A clean kill is all you need.' Says one attorney, 'Bower always reminds me of a German submarine captain.' "

Dan glanced up at me. "Listen to this part:

"The greatest challenge in his work, Bower says, is to represent vested corporate interests against badly injured individuals with solid cases. 'You have to humanize the defendant,' Bower instructs. 'I tried a trucking case once where the truck backed up and hit some guy, knocking out his teeth, fracturing his skull. He had all kinds of terrible problems. The plaintiff's demand was $150,000 or $200,000, and all I had to offer him from the insurance company was $37,500. It was tried in Queens with an essentially white picket fence jury. Now, the plaintiff and his eyewitness were slightly on the tender side, and the truck driver was a small 63-year-old Italian guy who looked like a miniature Fiorello LaGuardia, and his wife sat there in a black dress with no jewelry, holding his hand. Well, we made it a contest between the people—this nice old conservative Italian couple, and this rather swishy queen type. Of course, when you sum up, you never mention the trucking company, you talk about Angelo here—and it works.' Bower erupts in sudden, staccato laughter. 'The jury empathized, and accepted what was essentially a pretty poor defense story. We convinced them that the plaintiff was guilty of contributory negligence: he crossed behind the truck; he should've seen it backing up,' says Bower, breaking into laughter once more. 'They threw the case out of court. It's just got to be packaged right,' he stresses.

The people Bower turns out of court are often the blind, the brain damaged, and the maimed. Does he ever feel a surge of sympathy for these plaintiffs? 'Absolutely not,' Bower replies. 'My sympathies are not wasted on the enemy. Any plaintiff may have a meritorious lawsuit, but they're the enemy—it's that simple. My sympathies are reserved for the people who pay my fees.'

"Wait, Dick. You haven't heard anything yet," Dan assured me, with a hoarse harshness in his voice. "Talk about atrocities. This is the part that really blew my mind. A pig, italicized *pig*, he calls this poor woman:

"The plaintiff in the case was a 35-year-old black woman who had come to Joint Diseases with a condition doctors had diagnosed as cancer of the cervix. In opening up the patient, the doctors not only found evidence of pelvic inflammatory disease; they also inadvertently created a small hole, or fistula, between the patient's anus and vagina, 'so she had feces coming out of her vagina,' Bower explains. When they brought her to another hospital some months later, 'the doctors there accidentally tear the bladder, tear the gut, and they not only screw up her urethra but create a fistula between the bladder and the vagina, so she's leaking piss. Plus now she has an unrepairable, permanent colostomy. The bag.' Bower laughs. 'Great case to defend, isn't it?'

" 'She's okay on the cancer, though,' Bower resumes. 'My defense really ought to be . . .'—he pauses for effect—'that colostomy prevents metastasis.'

"In Bower's line of work, which includes a great deal of medical malpractice, cases like that of the woman with cancer and PID (pelvic inflammatory disease) come to seem almost ordinary, and defending the indefensible is just part of the job. But after the first day of trial on her case, Bower observed that the jury (to whom he had referred, when they were selected, as a 'panel of apes') 'visibly hated' his client. What upset him, however, was not so much that he thought the prognosis for the defendant was poor, but that the whole thing seemed so wrong. 'Everyone's been referring to her condition as PID,' he complained. 'No one's said it was neglected gonorrhea. But I certainly will.

" 'She's coming into court and asking to be made whole,' he

221

continued hotly. 'A promiscuous jerk who neglects her VD, a welfare mother of two illegitimate children—should we make her a millionaire? I say we could make her whole by giving her six cents—and some plastic bags.' "

If Dan's anger over the intimidation incident had reminded me of a sputtering fuse, this, then, was the explosion.

"Well?" he demanded, getting up to pace the study. 'You've been in the fray for a long time, have you ever heard anything like this? Isn't it the worst?"

I nodded. There was, of course, no doubt about that. "But what is diametrically opposed to the worst?"

"You're asking me riddles? The best, so?"

"Well, it helps to remember, that's all. If their side has John Bower, our side has Michael. And it has Marvin Ellin." For all the while Dan was reading defense lawyer Bower's story, I'd been thinking of his counterpart. If Bower thought of himself as an archcombatant sent out to battle, well, there were some excellent white knights he had to fight. And to my mind, and the minds of many grateful plaintiffs, Ellin is the best, compassionate with his clients and consummately skillful in the courtroom.

Dan stopped his pacing and sat down on the arm of the sofa, his fury spent at last. " 'Right must be defended against might, and the distressed must be protected,' " he quoted, reaching back into our schoolboy days to the Knights of the Round Table, with an embarrassed, self-mocking little smile.

"I was just thinking along these same lines myself," I confessed.

Dan took out his pipe, carefully filling it with his aromatic tobacco, packing it down so thoughtfully I doubted it would draw.

"You remember telling me once that you couldn't beat the system maybe but at least you could fight it?"

"Sure I do," I said. "Still feel the same way."

"Well, I've been thinking." Dan smiled. "For thirteen years, I guess, and that's long enough to be sitting on the sidelines. So what I came to say is, if somebody's been hurt, if there's an injured patient who needs a well-qualified cardiac surgeon to review the

222

files—well, will you and Paula tell them you know a guy who's willing?"

"Dan, old buddy, I thought you'd never ask," I said, laughing, but I guess I'm old enough, and man enough, to admit that there were tears in my eyes.